small
CHANGES

a **rules-free** guide to add more **plant-based** foods, **peace & power** to your life

ALICIA WITT

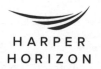

HARPER
HORIZON

Recipe testing by Donna Britt

Food photography by Tambi Lane

Professional portraits by Travis Commeau

All other photos provided courtesy of the author from her private collection

ISBN 978-0-7852-4032-7 (eBook)
ISBN 978-0-7852-4031-0 (HC)

Library of Congress Control Number: 2021939408

Printed in the United States of America

21 22 23 24 25 LSC 10 9 8 7 6 5 4 3 2 1

*For everyone along the way who has
inspired me to write this—every
conversation and connection—and for
everyone searching. This is for you.*

Contents

Introduction vii

Part I: How to Start Living Your Most Authentic Life

Chapter 1: Go Easy on Yourself—with Small Changes 2

Part II: The No-Rules Philosophy About Eating

Chapter 2: A (More) Plant-Based Lifestyle Is Easier Than You Think . . . 26

Chapter 3: Small Changes in Your Kitchen Give You Big Results 51

Chapter 4: "The Beans Do Not Exist": A Guide to
    Eating Away from Home 74

Part III: Caring for Your Mind, Spirit, and Soul

Chapter 5: Finding Your Way to a Healthy Inner Life 104

Chapter 6: Finding Yourself in the Silence 141

Part IV: Caring for Your Body

Chapter 7: Love Your Body—and Watch It Transform 162

Chapter 8: Small Changes to Your Lifestyle 177

Part V: The Recipes

Chapter 9: Small Changes Recipes 198

Part VI: The Exercises

Chapter 10: Low-Stress, Small Changes Exercises 252

Acknowledgments 264

Notes 266

About the Author 270

Introduction

Go on, you got this one life to live
You gotta take up your hook and sail

—"BLINKERS"

Deciding you want your life to be healthier, more balanced, and more connected is a big, big step.

Maybe you're motivated by your own unique health and fitness challenges, a work-life balance that isn't quite working for you, or a concern for the imprint you're leaving behind on the world. The question is: Once you've made the decision to change, where do you start? How will you know what to do without being consumed by rules, judgments, and restrictions? How can you live in a way that's respectful to others and to the world around you, while best serving your own well-being and still prioritizing a life that's authentic to how *you* want to live?

If you're anything like me, you've probably spent a lot of time thinking about these questions—especially when the guidance that experts offer in books, on TV, or online can be overwhelming. The truth is, you don't have to pay hundreds of dollars for meditation classes in order to be comfortable in your own mind, and you definitely don't need to join the most exclusive gym or fad-of-the-moment fitness class to have a healthy, strong, and fit body. If you choose to include more plant-based foods in your meals, you shouldn't feel like you have to abide by draconian rules that require you to empty your entire kitchen before you're accepted into the cult. No one gets to tell you what rules you live by—except for *you*!

If you want to improve your health, your consciousness, and the world, you don't need to overhaul your life in a drastic, overwhelming way. Sometimes all it takes are a few small changes to help you find your authenticity.

That's what this book is about.

Small Changes is a guide to help you find balance, eat better, and feel healthier physically and emotionally, and it offers a look at how I pull it all together as a successful actor, singer-songwriter, producer, rescue animal guardian, amateur farmer, homemade margarita aficionado—oh, and now author! Most importantly—and it's been a long road to this point—I've finally learned how to do it while staying deeply centered, even amidst chaos and uncertainty.

An Accidental Guru: Why Me and How This Book Came to Be

I've had such an odd career, but in a really cool way. I'm not so well-known that people chase me down the street, but whenever I go out, I get recognized. Given the wide range of diverse roles I've played over the span of my career, and the multitude of genres and projects I've been a part of, I'm almost always wrong if I try to guess the answer to that hilarious question working actors are asked constantly: "What have I seen you in?" (As you'll probably be relieved to know, I don't lurk in your living room, keeping tabs on your viewing history, and I haven't been spying on you over the years as you went to the movies.)

I live in Nashville now, and I find a sense of great peace when I'm in my vegetable garden, doing household chores, running errands at Home Depot, or spending time with my close-knit family of friends at one of our houses. Living such a "normal" day-to-day life when I'm not working also allows me to do better work on film or in a recording studio, or sitting alone writing a song or a screenplay, because everything else in my life is in balance.

That's my core philosophy in a nutshell: balance and authenticity. I'm not writing this book as an expert, because I'm far from that. I'm not a trained nutritionist. I'm not even a trained actor! I've never taken an acting class. I never attended public school. My only formal training thus far in my life has been as a classical pianist.

But, for whatever reason, I've become a kind of accidental guru.

∞∞∞∞∞∞∞∞∞∞∞

In 2003, I was in London to film the movie *The Upside of Anger*. The night after we all arrived for rehearsals, Keri Russell and I met up at The Ladbroke Arms in Notting Hill, a short walk from where we were staying. I was teaching Keri how to play backgammon at our table beneath the awning out on the patio, enjoying the perfect summer night, when a black cat suddenly was thrown out the window of the apartment above the pub. The cat bounced off the awning, and as it scrambled, claws outstretched, desperate to find its footing, it landed on my face and then raced away into the night.

"What *was* that?" I said to Keri. It was such a shock, like being slapped really hard in the face with something big and warm and heavy. I didn't register that something significant had happened until I saw the look on Keri's face. Touching my face, I realized how heavily I was bleeding. My upper lip was completely split in two.

In the ambulance, the EMT guy said, "Well, you know, scars give you character."

My head and heart were reeling. I was twenty-eight years old and at that point, I very much bought into the idea that as a female actor, your looks were synonymous with your career. We were about to start filming, and I was terrified not only that I would need to be replaced in this film, but that my livelihood as I knew it would be over.

But when our director, Mike Binder, joined us in the ER waiting room, he assured me, "I want you to know that no matter what, we're going to shoot around this. You're not going to lose the part." He was an actor himself—I loved him for understanding that this comparatively trivial thought was even in my head at that moment. After I'd thanked him through my tears, Mike thought about it for a little while and then said one of the funniest things I've ever heard: "Hey, at least you don't have to worry about *that* happening ever again." Cat falling from sky onto face: check!

That cat was actually the beginning of my journey toward being authentic. And strangely, even that night, I somehow understood it had happened for a reason. It was too utterly specific not to have been. Adding to the already bizarre scenario, a few years earlier my own (feral) cat had bitten me on the mouth, mere centimeters from this new injury. She'd missed splitting my lip by just-that-much, but the injury had required eight tiny stitches, so as to avoid leaving a scar right along the line of my philtrum. Though I couldn't yet work out what it was, I sensed that I'd missed the previous message, so the Universe delivered it to me again, with a lot more emphasis!

The next morning, Mike hooked me up with an expert plastic surgeon, and the stitches came out ten days after they went in—the morning I was scheduled to start filming. The makeup artist had achieved her certification concealing burns on people who'd been scarred in fires, so she was uniquely qualified to make the scratch invisible during shooting. As the wound healed, I was advised to wear makeup on it only while filming, and I had a bright red scar for months.

With the injury as my most noticeable feature, I recognized with humility that what I'd experienced up to that point in my life was the effortless attention that someone perceived as attractive receives on a daily basis. Going to Caffè Nero first thing in the morning and seeing the barista look directly at the cut across my upper mouth, instead of my eyes, as he said, "Can I take your order?" somehow helped me realize that what I had to offer the world—and myself— was about a lot more than my appearance. My purpose had to do with creative expression, communication, and personal peace. And I felt intense gratitude for the revelation.

From that moment on, I've thought about beauty differently. My scar has become one of my favorite features—while I remain grateful every day for that gifted surgeon who sewed my lip back together flawlessly. It healed so well it's visible only at certain angles or up close. I've always appreciated those who have looked at me deeply enough to notice it and ask me about it.

I clearly see that my life can be divided into before- and after-cat-scratch. My confidence has grown immensely, and I've been moving ever closer to living my authentic life, ever since I abandoned the notion that I should try to be some version of what others want me to be. Once I stopped worrying about my external appearance first and foremost, I feel I became a better actor, and I began writing consistently—and as a side result, I truly believe my external appearance improved too.

As I became more comfortable in my own skin, people noticed a certain energy in me. I never intended to be an accidental guru, but especially over the past ten years, I've had near-daily conversations with complete strangers. They approach me with all sorts of questions about things. Why I moved to Nashville, where I got the delicious-looking meal I'm eating that they couldn't find on any menu in the airport, what I'm wearing or using on my skin . . . or just how happy I seem to be! I'm the last person to say, "It's my way or the high- way," and my guess is that perhaps this is why people started finding it easy to ask me these sorts of questions, sensing they wouldn't receive a lecture. I get such joy from sharing a bit of insight from my own experiences with someone who's curious. And so I found myself talking regularly to people about small changes that might work for them.

Like Fran, my lovely Airbnb host when I was working on the ABC show *Nashville* in early 2016. Fran, who immediately felt like family—and is now part of my sacred inner circle of chosen family in Nashville—noticed the large portable jug I filled with water every day. Such a simple thing, but it had never occurred to her to use one—she and her dogs either drank tap water, or she bought single-use plastic bottles. She was not only barely hydrating herself but was wasting her money and creating trash when there was a store five minutes from her home that sold gallon refills of purified, alkaline water. So for a couple of dollars and a giant reusable jug, Fran got a constant supply of good-quality water. When she told me how this small change was instrumental in improving her own health as well as her dogs' health, I realized that these small changes weren't so small after all. They could have a *huge* impact! (Fran still uses and refills her jugs.)

This book evolved organically, as a result of experiences I've had with people like Fran. The philosophy at the heart of it is not a "start at square one and change your life drastically" plan. It's incremental.

My goal is for this book to help anyone who wants a change in their life, even those who may not know specifically *what* that change is—only that something's got to give. Maybe your health-care provider is saying you need to lower your cholesterol. Maybe you feel you don't have enough energy when you wake up in the morning. Maybe your body isn't functioning at what you know could be its peak potential. Maybe you want to find a little serenity. Maybe you just feel stuck.

Through my lines of work, I've met many different types of people, and almost everyone, wherever they live, has the same kinds of questions about finding their own authenticity and purpose in life. While I don't have all the answers, by sharing my experiences and offering practical advice and tips that have worked well for me, my hope is that I'll be able to help and inspire others to achieve their goals.

The Small Changes Philosophy

This book isn't about drastic or trendy diets, but it does illustrate how incorporating elements of my vegan food choices can make your meals healthier, without sacrificing taste or satisfaction. It won't prescribe tough workouts with expensive equipment or classes, but it will share some super-quick and effective at-home exercise routines that can fit into almost any schedule or lifestyle. It won't be about copying the way I meditate or emulating my day-to-day life, but rather how I hope my stories will help you find a routine that feels perfect for you—borrowing any or all of mine along the way! Regardless of what you want to improve, I hope you'll find guidance from my strategies and tools, and learn how small changes can usher in larger changes and transform your life.

My philosophy of small changes applies to everything. If you work out a little every day, for example, you'll get into the habit of working out, and you'll start feeling and seeing improvements, perhaps noticing you're enjoying life a bit more. Pretty soon you're drinking more water, living a healthier lifestyle, and feeling better in every possible way.

Research supports my belief that forming new habits works better when we start small. But rather than bog you down with statistics, I'll share my own unusual journey to health and happiness—through the incredible adventure my life has been thus far, and some of the extraordinary people I've met along that journey.

Small Changes is organized into six parts:

- In part I, "How to Start Living a More Authentic Life," I share my backstory, how I began this journey of small changes, my basic outlook on health and wellness, and how I came to write this book.
- Part II, "The No-Rules Philosophy About Eating," shows you how to easily incorporate a more plant-based diet into your life, small step by small step.

- In part III, "Caring for Your Mind, Spirit, and Soul," I'll suggest methods that have helped me develop and/or enhance my inner life and block out the noise, including meditation and journaling.
- Part IV, "Caring for Your Body," includes practical information about taking care of your body and making small, practical changes in your lifestyle.
- In part V, "The Recipes," you'll find some of my favorite original recipes that are easy, inexpensive, and delicious!
- Finally, part VI, "The Exercises," includes the short and simple exercise routine I do at home and when I'm on the road. My routine keeps me in shape and fills me with the energy I need to keep my metabolism up, even when I don't have much time—and I bet it'll help do the same for you.

To quote Jon Kabat-Zinn's book title: *Wherever you go, there you are.* I am the one constant that I know. I've learned to be content and happy and peaceful in my own company, not defined by my work or my appearance or any of my relationships. And it's all due to the small changes I made that turned into big ones that have transformed my life.

I want you to love the changes you'll make—to not only feel better, but to be excited about making them. Start small, enjoy the learning curve, discover what aspects of this book resonate for you, and embrace them. Love yourself, whatever you're doing. Your choices are uniquely your own, and each person is their own small-changes ambassador. You don't have to preach to change the world: lead by example—and watch what happens!

PART I

How to Start Living Your Most

authentic life

CHAPTER 1

Go Easy on Yourself— with Small Changes

Hold your head up high to face the past

—"JUDGMENT DAY"

Where does authenticity come from?

In show business, you hear a lot about "big breaks," but my story as an actor and a musician has been fueled and sustained by many small changes over the years. And for me, it starts with the notion of being easy on yourself.

Whether with work, relationships, food, exercise, skincare, getting stuff done, or even goofing off, the principle is the same: treating yourself (and others) with kindness—even if you mess up sometimes!—will lead to the small changes that eventually turn into the big changes you seek. If you can come to this understanding, you'll feel better, reflect better energy from the inside out, and achieve improved overall happiness.

So let me take you back to the beginning, and the unusual trajectory of my life.

Dune, Piano, and Learning to Cook: The Early Years

I was born in 1975 in Worcester, Massachusetts. I had an unorthodox upbring-ing, to put it mildly. Homeschooling is much more commonplace now—even more so since the COVID-19 pandemic—but in those days it was almost unheard of. However, that's the only school experience I've ever had. I became advanced beyond my years in some ways, while entirely skipping over the typical child-hood routine of school, playdates, and sports activities. We weren't allowed to watch much TV either, so my brother and I became proficient at Monopoly, cribbage, and chess, and created elaborate stories—complete with family trees tracing lineage and histories—with our dollhouses and the miniature people who inhabited them. We lived in our own little universe.

My father was a brilliant science teacher, and my mother had been a junior high school reading specialist before she decided to stay at home full-time after I was born. She started teaching me to read when I was a baby, and I was read-ing fluently by the time I was three. After she sent a letter to the editor of *Good Housekeeping*, including a photo of me reading their magazine, they ran a story about their "youngest reader." This led to my appearance on several vari-ety shows, including *That's Incredible!*, which featured people with unusual skills. When I was five, they flew my family and me out to LA, and I performed the balcony scene from *Romeo and Juliet* in front of an audience—my first time experiencing such a thing. I loved being onstage, and parting was such sweet sorrow! (And we got to go to Disneyland the next day too.)

As fate would have it, two years later casting director Jane Jenkins was searching for an advanced child to play the role of Alia in the sci-fi film *Dune*. (For those of you unfamiliar with the David Lynch adaptation of the Frank Herbert novel, Alia was born with the knowledge of generations of Reverend Mothers before her—a four-year-old with an adult vocabulary.) After months of searching with no luck, Jane decided to call *That's Incredible!* in case they knew of some child with extraordinary verbal skills, and they sent her a VHS tape of my segment. She got my parents' number, and soon we were on our way to New York City for me to audition—first for her, then for David Lynch. I still clearly remember that audition, as within five minutes of first meeting David, I regaled him with tales of all the different dogs who lived on my street—which he recently reminded me of while working together for a fourth time on *Twin Peaks*. Then he gave me direction on the three scenes I'd been asked to prepare.

Later that week I told my parents, "I think I'm going to get that part." Sure enough, I was cast. I turned eight during the shoot, and being there was the best birthday present I could have ever received! I knew from the first moment I set foot on the set that I wanted to act for the rest of my life, and consequently started imploring my parents to let me move to LA.

Understandably, my parents didn't want to immediately uproot the family. Besides, I'd started taking piano lessons when I was seven, and after only a few weeks it became obvious that I was taking to it in a big way. Because I loved playing so much, I practiced for hours every day and eventually was taking four lessons a week. It may sound like a lot, but especially since I wasn't attending school or participating in any group activities, it makes sense to me. Kids who play sports are often with the team for hours most days after school, and they don't see it as a chore because they're doing something they love. And the more I learned on the piano, the more I loved it. After less than a year of lessons, I competed in my first classical competition, and I won. I was soon racking up ribbons and trophies.

This is where my unusual upbringing was a plus, because if I'd been going to public school, I probably would've gotten interested in many other things. Instead, the piano became something I poured everything I had into, and it also became an outlet for me. Not just because I loved playing but because when I went to recitals or competitions, I could interact with kids my age, which was fun.

I started playing dinner background music in a restaurant when I was ten, which helped pay for all the lessons. I played all the classical pieces I knew, as well as my dad's favorite pop songs and the big band music of his generation. (Nat King Cole is still one of my absolute all-time favorites.) So I built up a sizeable repertoire of songs and show tunes that you might hear in a piano bar.

That's the music of my childhood, as though I'd grown up in the 1940s; to me, those songs sound like what songs should be. I hear the beginning refrain to a tune from that era, and I still know all the words—while to this day I'm unfamiliar with much of what would've been considered "cool" for a kid to listen to growing up in the eighties. I was like an old musical fuddy-duddy as a child!

But even then I knew that becoming a professional classical pianist was not my heart's calling. I had a vague vision of who I'd be when I grew up: I saw myself making my own music and playing my own songs. And acting, of course.

That vision became clearer when *That's Incredible!* scheduled a reunion show when I was twelve. They again flew my family and me out to LA, and as our plane circled over the city and I saw it below me, I had this overwhelming, inexplicable feeling that this was where I was supposed to be living. Where my destiny was waiting for me.

We were only there for three days, but my mom got in touch with David Lynch, and he invited us to his house. Somehow I got to talking about music with him, and he told me how he liked to listen to it really loud, which contradicted what my mother had told me: that music should be quietly listened to, so you didn't hurt your ears.

"Not for me," David said. "You have to turn it up so you can really lose yourself inside of it."

I remember that moment vividly, because it changed the way I thought about music.

After that trip I started full-on begging my parents to help me get back to LA to try to secure an agent, so I could go for acting in earnest. I'd auditioned for and gotten cast in one film shooting in Boston when I was ten, but funding fell through after I'd been on set one day, and it never finished. And two other auditions had come my way from having been in *Dune*. But I knew there was no way I could pursue an acting career if I lived in Worcester.

Fortunately, when I was thirteen, I qualified for an international piano competition held at UCLA, and that meant my mother and I would need to be in LA for several weeks. While we were there, I had some meetings and was signed by my first agent, who started setting up acting auditions. They set me up to have some photos taken for modeling as well, but I didn't get any work there. I was awkward, understandably, and modeling is so objective. In retrospect, I'm grateful I didn't end up getting into that world. Also, not knowing any other teenagers meant I was an unusual mix of very mature and very immature, which didn't help at the modeling casting calls, where even thirteen-year-olds were expected to be more womanly than young-girlish.

My mom and I ended up moving to LA for seven months when I was fourteen. We stayed in a hotel the entire time—the then-Holiday Inn on Wilshire Boulevard in Westwood—because we weren't sure how long we'd be there, but it was expensive. To help pay for it, I played piano occasionally in the lobby bar downstairs, and during Sunday brunch at what was then the Westwood Marquis (now the W Hotel). When I was at those gigs, I'd pick up other jobs, playing background music at private events, like birthday parties at fancy homes.

Still, I knew I'd need more money to be able to afford to stay. When watching *Wheel of Fortune* one night, I learned they were holding auditions—in LA—for the first-ever prime-time version of Teen Week. (The daytime syndicated episodes were half the money value on the wheel!) After five rounds of mock games, written tests, and a final interview, I was selected to be one of fifteen contestants that week. I was excited because I knew I was good at the game, so there was real potential for me to earn money that could meaningfully keep me in LA for a while. As it turned out, I hit bankrupt twice, but I did win $2,700, which was something! And when Pat Sajak asked me about myself, I proudly answered (in my Worcester accent and lisp) that I was an actor and a musician. He replied, deadpan: "Well, I'm glad you could take time out of your busy schedule to be here with us tonight." Eight years later, when I appeared on Celebrity Week (and won big, for a charitable donation), they played that clip.

During this same time, David Lynch wrote the role of Gersten Hayward for me on *Twin Peaks*, which was a huge blessing because suddenly, I had a recent credit on one of the most acclaimed and talked-about shows on TV. Not only did this help get me in the door for auditions, but weirdly, it also got me a high school "diploma" at age fourteen!

When I was hired for *Twin Peaks*, a minor on set couldn't legally have their teacher and their guardian be the same person—which in my case, of course, was my mom. A few phone calls later, the Worcester superintendent of schools, a family friend, faxed over a statement saying I'd completed my education through grade twelve. In an unheard-of situation even back then, I wasn't officially tested. I've never taken my SATs or GEDs. Just between us! (Oh wait . . .)

Around that time, I was standing in the lobby of the Beverly Wilshire Hotel when I noticed a man staring intently at me. Which sounds creepy, but quickly wasn't once he came over and introduced himself to me (and my mom) as director Mike Figgis. He told me there was a small role as a girl who may or may not be real in a movie called *Liebestraum*, which he was going to start filming—and he thought I might be right for it (not knowing that I'd acted before). When I told him I played piano, we went into the restaurant off the lobby, which was nearly empty, and I played a few songs on that piano. He then explained that his movie was named after "Liebestraum," Liszt's famous piano composition, and if I could learn it in time, he'd put it in the movie. I got the sheet music and learned it over the next few months, and you can see me as the "Girl in Dream" playing it during the end credits.

"Liebestraum" has become the piece I always play first to become familiarized with a new piano—in a recording studio, on a set where I'm about to perform in character, or to ease my nerves in a nonmusical setting, if there happens to be a piano around. *Liebestraum* means "dream of love." I love that piece with all my heart. It sounds not only like it could be the act of lovemaking from beginning to end, but it could be the musical description of a dream where you're imagining a love that doesn't exist, or a love gone by. Or it can even be an entire life itself, from start to finish. It's such a phenomenally gorgeous song.

After filming *Liebestraum* in New York, the plan had been for me to move back to LA with my mom, but her parents' health was failing, so we returned to Worcester for another year and a half to be with my grandparents until they passed away. I was able to keep auditioning in New York, and the role I got closest to was in *Cape Fear.* After several callbacks, it was down to me and Juliette Lewis at the final audition, acting opposite Robert De Niro, with Martin Scorsese directing—not that I had the faintest clue at that time how extraordinary it was to be in a room working with those two! Although I learned how disappointing it could be to get *thaaaat close* and not be the one chosen for such a huge job, I could see, even at age fifteen, that it was a sign I was on the right track. I knew for sure I wasn't crazy to be thinking I might have a future in the industry, and I was encouraged to know that I'd *almost* gotten the role.

Learning from failure or disappointment is an important part of trusting yourself to make the changes you need to make.

Sometimes, the thing that's meant for you will find you on its own time.

You just have to keep faith, do great work, and wait your turn. It all comes down to how badly you want it and how much you believe in yourself. This has been one of my greatest life lessons over the years.

Fun Changed My Life

I was able to move back to LA with my mom when I was sixteen, and I got a job as a pianist two, then three, then five nights a week in the lobby lounge of the Regent Beverly Wilshire Hotel. I wasn't partying or drinking or dating or . . . anything! I was just there to make my mark. During the day, I sometimes went on as many as three auditions: for commercials, tiny roles, one episode of something, big roles, you name it. I'd take the bus around town with my hair under a baseball cap, wearing baggy and nondescript clothes so I wouldn't attract unwanted attention. I made sure I arrived at my appointment early enough to change into my cute meeting outfit and fluff out my hair in the restroom, then I'd change back again before walking to the bus stop. I'd hurry to the Beverly Wilshire for my gig; if you were two minutes late, they gave you the evil eye. (I still have recurring dreams about showing up late to that gig, or falling asleep in the employees' lounge and realizing with a start that I've taken way too long of a break. Thirty years later!)

That year's auditions were one frustration after another. Classical musicians' brains are shaped by their rigorous training, and the discipline and nerves of steel I'd acquired performing onstage in competitions became invaluable when I went on acting auditions and, later, during the filming of challenging scenes. But along with navigating the uncharted waters of LA's entertainment scene, I had to learn how to take care of myself.

One of the best things that came out of that year was learning to manage the multitasking that I've gotten so good at. I had to quickly switch from the mode of whatever characters I was auditioning for into logistical mode, to figure out how much time I had after the last audition to make it to the hotel, so I could be sitting on that piano bench at exactly 4:00 p.m.

I was also aware of what a blessing playing piano for a living was. I was tremendously grateful I could support myself with the skill I'd worked so hard to build—even though on a daily basis I was faced with well-meaning patrons who'd ask me what my plans were, assuming I was planning to study at a conservatory. When I told them why I was in LA, they'd wince in dismay and reply, "Oh no, you don't want to do that. This town is full of actresses—you should be a pianist. You're *really* good at this!" I'd smile while bristling inside, thinking, *Well, you don't know this yet, but I'm a good actor too.* Some days it felt like I was expending most of my mental energy trying to prove everyone wrong.

And then a beautiful thing, a turning-point marker in life, happened.

On one of these nights, the director Rafael Zielinski was in the hotel for a meeting. He watched me play, and similarly to what had happened with Mike Figgis at the same hotel, Rafael approached me and said he had a script he was looking to film in the next few months. He asked if I'd ever considered acting, because he had a feeling I could be right for this part. Not having seen the few things I'd acted in up to that point, he was pleasantly surprised to hear I wasn't a novice at it.

The movie was called *Fun*, loosely based on a true story of two teenagers in Northern California who murdered an elderly woman, both insisting afterward that the sole motive was "fun." The character I auditioned for, Bonnie, was a fibber who would go on and on at the speed of light, like this whirling dervish of energy who was clearly not well. But she was so entertaining and full of life that you wanted to love her—except, of course, when she made the dubious choice to stab a random elderly lady forty-seven times! It was a challenging and complicated role, and I longed to play her as soon as I read it. I was elated when Rafael offered me the part, even though the whole thing had a bit of an experimental vibe, with a super-low budget to match.

It was intense work. We had a mind-blowingly brief seven days in which to film *the entire movie*, and we rehearsed and rehearsed the long scenes and the extensive dialogue, so by the time the shoot started, we knew we'd be able to nail it in the few takes we'd have. We had a waiver from the Screen Actors Guild so we could work much longer than union hours, and there wasn't any time to get out of character in between driving home from set and heading back to work. For that week I lived and breathed my character—and I ended up having very disturbing dreams. The prison scenes were filmed at the LA detention center for youths, so we often saw actual prisoners my age who were real-life killers. We had permission to film there, but there were other locations where we didn't, and Rafael would grab a shot before we got chased away. It was surreal, to say the least, and we were astonished when the film was chosen for the Sundance Film Festival.

In January 1994 I attended Sundance, and everywhere I went people had seen the movie and were complimenting me. I couldn't believe it. It almost felt as though I'd landed in some alternate universe where I was a well-known actor. Then my costar, Renée Humphrey, and I were stunned to receive a Special Jury Recognition for Acting award at the closing ceremony—the first time the festival had given an acting award. When I heard my name called, I thought I'd lost my mind! I was giddy at the thought that I'd actually make a living at this thing I'd been wanting to prove I could do for as long as I could remember. It was the first time anyone had officially said I was good at this. Not only did I *not* need to go to Juilliard and be a classical piano player, but I now had an acting award to prove it.

I was in such a state that when I got on stage to accept (alone—Renée had skipped the ceremony, since we had no reason to think we'd get an award), I forgot to thank Rafael or anybody associated with the movie. Grasping at straws from what I'd seen watching the Oscars over the years, the only people I could think to thank were my agent, manager, and publicist. I was *so* embarrassed afterward! Especially when *Variety* mentioned my horrible acceptance speech in their Sundance wrap-up. But, as I realized once I got over the shame of being called out for my first big public faux pas, at least they mentioned it!

Fun changed the trajectory of my career. It hadn't paid enough for me to quit my piano playing job, but instead of going on three auditions a day for commercials and tiny parts, I started meeting on all the major roles for girls my age, and casting directors started bringing me in to meet with the directors without having to read for them first. I got a pretty big role in a CBS movie of the week, and right before I left for Vancouver to film it, I had the opportunity to audition for *Mr. Holland's Opus.*

Then I had to learn the song "Stranger on the Shore" on the clarinet; they gave me a month of lessons, and I practiced diligently until I could play it flawlessly. (It's much easier to learn a new instrument when you can already play another.) But when I played it for the music supervisor upon arriving in Portland, he said, "Wow—that's perfect. The only problem is you're supposed to be really bad at it!" So I had to take a few more lessons to learn how to squeak on cue!

Not only was *Mr. Holland's Opus* a movie about music, but far more important to me was that my dad had been a teacher all his life and had just retired, so it resonated deeply. I was honored to be a part of it. Filming those scenes with Richard Dreyfuss—who was truly respectful of my work and treated me as a colleague, even though I was such an unknown—it felt like all that mattered was what my character was experiencing. The genuine sense of becoming Gertrude, with all her insecurity and transformation, made me even more determined to keep acting.

The College of Cybill

The truth is, I wasn't ever seeking to do a sitcom, because the movies I'd always been close to getting, or the things I did get, were more dark and indie in sensibility. I'd never had a sitcom audition that led to a single callback, and I had decided to stop trying out for them. I wasn't a bright and sunny, commercially comedic sort of performer by nature, and that's what I thought sitcoms required. So *Cybill* became a beautiful example of how sometimes you don't know what's meant for you until it happens.

When I was first asked to audition, I didn't see how I was even physically right to play Zoey, the teenage daughter of quintessential blonde Cybill Shepherd. But my manager told me they were looking for Zoey not necessarily to be what you'd expect Cybill's daughter to look like—and that the comedy should be sarcastic and deadpan—so it was worth a shot. I did my thing and immediately got a callback (within an hour). The next audition was in a bigger room with some of the producers. I could tell it went well, which again surprised me.

Casting is always a bit of strange energy, because you have to put the seriousness of the potential at hand out of your mind. Focus on the scene; focus on what you intended to do. And enjoy playing that character because you never know—it might be the one and only time you ever play that role, if you don't get cast. This all adds to your mental gymnastics, when you're trying to not be nervous or intimidated by the sight of twenty people staring at you while you're hoping to be funny, or fun, or endearing, or whatever the character is. It's up to you to go in and do what you do and not croak, while a decision that might change your entire life rests on your performance. No pressure!

I also was falling in love with the character by this point, because the darker I played her, the more I made them laugh, and I hadn't seen a sitcom character like that before. Then I got another callback with all of the producers, the writers, and Cybill, so they could gauge our chemistry as mother and daughter. That went really well, and I realized that we could look like we were related—that there was something familiar in a family-sort-of-way about her. What I didn't realize at the time was that they'd already gone through this casting process four different times. They'd seen all the blondes who "looked like" Cybill, and when I finally came in, they were auditioning people they hadn't considered before.

For my final callback, all the network execs were there too. Afterward, I was walking into the parking garage at CBS when I heard a voice behind me call my name. I turned around, and it was Cybill.

"You got it, honey!" she said.

This experience taught me so much about fate. I know that many of the people who auditioned at that time were disappointed they didn't get the part. But I think the reason was that I was supposed to play Zoey, and they were supposed to have other roles—just as I've been gutted not to have been chosen for certain jobs that were someone else's destiny. This has become part of my religion at this point.

Finally, after the pilot episode was filmed and the show was picked up for its first season, I was able to quit my job at the Beverly Wilshire, where I had played for almost two and a half years. I would have a guaranteed significant paycheck for the first time in my life. When I wrote my two weeks' notice letter, I felt triumphant, knowing that all those years of telling people *I'm an actor* were finally proven true.

When the producers discovered I could play the piano, they decided Zoey would too. In Zoey's first scene in the first episode, she's playing the most complicated part of (what else?) "Liebestraum," yet the instant Cybill walks in the front door, Zoey abruptly slouches and switches to "Chopsticks" played with two fingers. Before I'd said a word, you already *knew* this character and what the mother-daughter dynamic was.

I learned so much when I was on *Cybill*—the experience of feeling like I was part of a group, almost as if those four years were my college years. When I started, I hadn't yet become comfortable with people my own age, whose life experiences seemed so alien to mine, but I grew close to the rest of the cast, who were all much older than me.

I still think of Alan Rosenberg, who played my dad, as my *other* dad. Incredibly compassionate and politically active, he taught me about looking deeper at people and situations, with love and without any judgment. I realized that, while I was extremely opinionated, many of my ideas were uninformed by actual life experience. He also taught me how to play backgammon, which became one of my absolute lifelong favorite pastimes. We'd play for money (fifty cents a point), and Alan was so proud of me because at the end of the final show, he owed me $400— and he'd been the New York State backgammon champion in 1981!

I also loved working with Christine Baranski, who brought such joy, laughter, and timeless class to the set. When she began working on the show, she was already well respected on Broadway and a two-time Tony winner, but unknown to TV and movie audiences. It was inspiring to watch her become this glamorous, instantly recognizable household name overnight, and to watch the fun she had with that. She set a terrific example of how to celebrate and embrace success while staying centered. It never changed who she was at her core; her true identity was at home in Connecticut with her family. And I was privileged to become close to them as well. That taught me so much about what really matters: that all the acclaim in the world means nothing if you don't know where—and who—home is.

Dedee Pfeiffer, who played my sister, became the big sister I'd never had in real life, and she was always a touchstone I could count on no matter what. She was also instrumental in teaching me how to be safe and protect myself. Everything shifted fast once *Cybill* started airing every week, because back then there were only four networks (no cable or streaming series), and the viewership for any successful show was enormous. Some security issues popped up pretty quickly, and I was grateful to have a mentor like Dedee to give me a crash course in what I needed to do to keep safe. Not to mention all the other rites of passage that a big sister would be there for! I also met my first boyfriend, Peter Krause, on the show, and we dated for three years. He played Dedee's husband, so "Does your sister know about this?" was a common query when we'd go out together.

It's not a secret, though, that *Cybill* became a difficult set to work on. Blisteringly smart and utterly unafraid, Zoey's personality was such that when everyone around her was putting on a happy face, she was the one who told it like it was. *She* didn't worry about being polite, and I appreciated that about her, as it made the role a lot of fun for me. Especially when times got tough on set, I had a blast playing a character who was wickedly sarcastic.

One big thing I learned (albeit, in retrospect) was what *not* to react to—a valuable skill in any career or facet of life. On subsequent sets, too, I've worked with challenging personalities. Having had that formative experience on *Cybill* for four years, and seeing the contrast between people who let the problems wash away versus people who allowed them to sink into their psyche, was invaluable. I now feel secure enough to get along with almost anybody at work.

I also started getting offers, or "offers pending a meeting with the director," for big movies, most of which I was unavailable for, since I was only free to film when we were on our three-month summer hiatus. It was confusing because I loved being on the show and I loved my friends on the set, but I missed the challenge of immersing myself in a new character.

Additionally, the financial security was astonishing. My dad had been the sole provider for our family, and we'd always had little money. I felt an incredible sense of pride to be able to buy him a car and fly him to LA for visits. I couldn't believe that I was making enough money to support myself and save up until I could eventually buy a house. Finances are something I've never taken for granted, and I was *so* grateful.

An Actor's Life

The day after we taped our final episode of *Cybill*, I left for Toronto to film *Urban Legend*, my first lead in a studio movie. That was a *very* big job for me, because I'd had many experiences of getting close to a lead role in a studio film and not being cast. I spent two and a half months in Toronto, running in the rain and screaming. (More about this experience in chapter 7.)

My next film was *Playing Mona Lisa*, which was another leading role. It had a much smaller budget, but from the beginning, everything about it felt uniquely magical. The character was written as a ballerina (a skill I only pretend to possess at late-night dance parties when I'm channeling my inner Jim Carrey), and when I suggested they change her to a classical pianist instead, they didn't think twice. That wonderful decision allowed me to incorporate my complicated relationship with the piano into this character—classical piano was part of me and would be forever, but it wasn't meant to be my career.

At the same time, my relationship with Peter was in the process of ending, which I didn't want to acknowledge yet, and I was dealing with the series having ended as well. It felt like graduating from college in a way, because I was on my own again. What helped me grow was to be on this set with actors who—and this is a rare experience—became friends for life. It was a community of such love and collaboration. I would go to work every day on cloud nine to be around these people, including Harvey Fierstein, who was such a beam of light. It felt like what I was *supposed* to be doing.

Playing Mona Lisa was also my first time playing the lead in something so lighthearted and comedic. I had so much fun becoming Claire. She was very similar to who I was in real life at that time, making the movie almost a personal time capsule. When people come up to me, maybe two or three times a year, and tell me this largely unknown film is their favorite movie, I get all teary-eyed.

The most valuable lesson I learned from working with this cast on that movie was, by contrast, that you can't expect everyone you meet or work with to be a tribe member. That's more than okay—that's the way it's supposed to be. A lot of peace comes from accepting this, and going to work to do the best you can and to collaborate with those who will make the project as good as it can be—and have fun doing it, hopefully. I know it's much the same no matter what you do for a living.

As the years continued, I worked steadily in television, movies, and theater. There were some lean seasons, which happens to many actors, and some crazy-busy ones. I guest-starred on *Ally McBeal* and *The Sopranos*, spent half a season on *Law and Order: Criminal Intent*, and recently I've been on *The Walking Dead*, the revival of *Twin Peaks*, and *Orange Is the New Black*. I've made countless films—big studio-financed movies like *Two Weeks Notice* and *Last Holiday*, ultra-low-budget indies, and everything in between—for big and small screens alike, including the enormous blessing that has been Hallmark Christmas movies. When I made my first one, *A Very Merry Mix-Up*, in 2013, I had no idea that they would become an annual gift. But I did know it was one of those sets that felt like angel dust was sprinkled over the entire process. I think you can see it in the movie too.

The Music in Me

Through Dedee, my *Cybill* sister, I met singer-songwriter Jude Cole. He was starting to produce and manage other artists, and I told him I wrote my own songs. After I played them for him, he wanted to explore collaborating. We made a demo of a song I wrote called "Purgatory," based on the melancholy I felt finishing *Playing Mona Lisa*, and we worked on a handful of others too.

A few months later, Jude said, "You know, I just don't think you're ready yet. I think you have a lot of stories to tell, but you need to write every day and figure out what it is you want to say and what your style is. Let's pick this back up in a year or so and see where you are then."

I was *devastated*. Looking back, I know he was right—he never said I was no good or that the songs were awful and I should quit. But I was so discouraged that I stopped writing songs for years and years. Instead, I'd play the classical music I knew so well, and it became almost a party trick kind of thing. I'd whip out a Chopin ballade and play it flawlessly and leave people impressed.

The turning point for my music came when a five-and-a-half-year relationship was coming to an end. I had finally come around to understanding that, although he was a truly great person, he wasn't *my* person. He wasn't the one I was supposed to spend the rest of my life with. The moment he moved out and closed the front door behind him, I was flooded with such a wave of relief and of authenticity that I sat down at the piano and started to write. That was in December 2006, and I haven't stopped writing since.

In a way, ending that relationship was the biggest decision I'd ever made— one that came purely from my heart and my instincts, and not because anything I could put my finger on was wrong. I knew I had more to do, and without being able to describe it at the time, I also knew those songs were waiting to be born, and they weren't going to come out if I stayed in that relationship. I needed to ascend to a new level of fearlessness and freedom.

The song I started writing that day is called "Blind," and it's on my first EP that I released in 2009. Almost every day since, I've written *something*. It took all of those years for me to figure out what it was I wanted to say, without even knowing I was figuring it out. Once I started, I couldn't stop and the ideas were flowing, one after another. At any given time, I have maybe five unfinished songs dancing around my head, waiting for the right moment to be finished. I'll write some lyrics before I go to bed and some more when I wake up. Or sometimes I'll complete the song in one flow, in only a few hours. And some of my songs have been started and completed years apart!

Music became an even more important part of my career when I moved to Nashville. I'd first visited in 2009 when my EP came out, and a friend invited me to open for him at this little songwriter gig. The Nashville of 2009 was very different than the Nashville of today—it was a lot smaller and less glamorous, but I had an indescribable feeling that it was where I belonged, much as I had felt about LA all those years earlier. I found my eyes unexpectedly brimming with tears as my plane took off the next day, but I didn't yet understand why.

Three years later I booked a songwriters' round at the Bluebird Cafe with songwriter Jeff Cohen (whom I'd met on that first visit to Nashville!), as part of my ten-city tour to celebrate the release of my album *Live at Rockwood*. Earlier on the day of the show, Jeff had set me up to write with his friend James Slater, and we grabbed lunch at the deli Noshville. As fate would have it, acclaimed singer-songwriter Ben Folds was sitting at the next table. Ben was working around the corner at his studio—RCA Studio A, where "Jolene" and many other classic songs were recorded—on his reunion album with his band, Ben Folds Five. We talked for a long time and then wrote a few songs remotely, he in Nashville and me in LA. I met other people during that brief trip and on the trips that followed. One thing led to another, and I started spending many months of every year in Nashville.

Ben and I dated for two years, and he produced and played multiple instruments on my record *Revisionary History*. We cowrote a duet (for my movie *Cold Turkey*) that's on the album, and another song we'd written, "I'm Not the Man," ended up on one of his albums. Every visit to Nashville was filled with writing sessions and meetings and recording. I had found a place where I felt at home, more than any other place I'd ever been. It didn't have to do with any particular person or connection—it was that same feeling I'd had on my first visit, as though some geographical conjunction was calling me back.

Being cast on the show *Nashville* in 2016 was another major turning point. I needed a place to stay, so I entered an incredibly narrow radius on Airbnb in the hopes that I'd find exactly what I wanted, and the first listing that popped up was from a woman named Fran (the same one I mentioned in the introduction!). When Ernest, my rescue dog, and I went to see the place in person, she and I talked for an hour as though we'd known each other forever. Then she called her best friend, Paula, and told her she'd met someone who she believed would be significant in their lives. She was right! Paula is now one of my best friends, and she also became extremely pivotal in my musical life. As a former music manager, she knew an incredible network of people, and she introduced me to amazing writers and producers. Her championing of me meant a lot at that specific moment. That combined with my work on *Nashville*—a show that everyone in town knew you couldn't get cast on unless you could really sing—changed the type of writing sessions I had.

Everything was falling into place in terms of my music; I was improving and growing as a writer and an artist. Beyond that, the turning point was the chosen family I'd found. And the more I accepted that I was peaceful and at home whenever I was in Nashville, the more I started feeling the inspiration I needed all around me.

Around this time I became drawn to crystals, especially blue kyanite, for reasons I couldn't exactly explain. I started wearing one as a necklace, and a few months after I met Paula, she brought me to a house party. A gal named Eliza Ann came up to me and asked about my blue kyanite, which she'd spotted across the room; it was also one of her favorites! Eliza Ann has become another of my absolute closest sister-friends. (I believe that's partially why I was drawn to wearing a blue kyanite in the first place. I still love it but no longer feel the need to wear it every day.) Even though I had close friends in LA, my community of incredible women in Nashville gave me a feeling of home that I'd never had anywhere else.

> Sometimes you can keep on doing what you're doing and be comfortable. But the creativity that's going to be unleashed when you make a small change can be so much more soul-satisfying.

All of this made me realize, by contrast, that I was falling out of love with LA. I no longer had to worry about being based there for work opportunities; the acting business had changed, and instead of in-person meetings, directors and producers often asked to see a filmed audition that actors could make themselves and send in, if they weren't in town to tape with the casting director. By 2017, I was admitting to myself that living in LA no longer felt authentic. Like the feeling you get sometimes when you're in a relationship that's not working, and you introduce them to someone as your partner, and something in you kind of jars.

Once I'd made the decision, I put my house on the market, and the exact same week I received two offers on it, a house popped up in Nashville that seemed perfect in its online listing. After taking a virtual tour, I made an offer—and it was accepted! I was about to head to Vancouver for three months to film a Christmas movie and the series *The Exorcist*, so I flew to Nashville, checked out the house in person, and made the decision to officially go forward with the purchase. Then I went to Vancouver for the first job, closed on my house in LA and moved out all my stuff, and then went back to Canada to start job number two.

As with all life decisions, of course you can't help wondering sometimes what would have happened had you done something sooner, but I see my life as being exactly the way it's supposed to be; I learned lessons I wouldn't have otherwise. Not a day goes by that I don't think moving to Nashville was one of the best decisions I've ever made, second only to my decision to move to LA when I was a teenager. In fact, gratitude that I live in Nashville is usually one of my first conscious thoughts when I wake up in the morning.

One of the most important things I've learned about is flexibility. I think it's an underrated word in a way. Having the courage of your convictions and bending like a tree in the wind, as opposed to standing there yelling *stop*. A key part of my philosophy now is that there are a million signs out there for all of us—we need only start paying attention to them. They'll tell us what is right, what resonates in our gut as true. They'll also tell us when it's time to embrace changes. Even small changes.

You have to be flexible if you're an actor—you're always playing different characters in different stories, with different people acting alongside you, different energies working together on the production as a team. You have to be flexible as a songwriter because writing a good song is often a process of endless revisions, and if you aren't willing to be flexible to the changes you need to make—open to what could be better—you're sealing yourself off from listening to your intuition and identifying when something isn't yet right. (Or when it's already right!)

Nurturing your own flexibility is a small change you can make that will turn into a very big change in how you respond to people and situations in your life. It's what led me to create my whole small changes philosophy—and to write this book.

So read on, and in the next few chapters you'll see how I adapted small changes to one of my favorite topics: food!

PART II

The No-Rules Philosophy

about eating

CHAPTER 2

A (More) Plant-Based Lifestyle Is Easier Than You Think

What if you're seeing it wrong and nothing was lost
We all have to make mistakes

—"THEME FROM PASADENA"

Imagine a world where, instead of eating red or processed meat two or three times a day—which is unhealthy and contributing to the epidemic of global warming and lack of food worldwide[1]—those who wish to eat meat ate it once a day. Or five times a week. Think about this: the United Nations Food and Agricultural Organization has reported that livestock produce 14.5 percent of all *global* greenhouse gas emissions.[2] That's a lot of hot air!

What if we lived in a world where, instead of abiding by labels and having to be either "vegan/vegetarian," or eating anything and everything that is available to us, we were gently, self-compassionately mindful of these choices? What if, instead of buying the cheapest meat available, we cut back and spent that money instead on organic, vegetarian-fed meat, supplementing our diets with filling, nutrient-rich, and less expensive protein sources?

Our meat sources would vastly improve. Livestock would have much more room to graze, and there would be less demand for mass production but more demand for high-quality meats—which would entail better lives for the animals, a better food source for you, and, I believe, a better world.[3]

Along with a positive, forgiving mindset, one of the most fundamental changes you can make in your life is incorporating healthier options into your diet. What you eat can affect your mood, your appearance, your energy level, and your mental health. For many people hoping to make small changes in their life, rethinking what you eat is one of the best places to start.

This is why I want to share with you how I came to live a mostly vegan lifestyle. From both an ethical and nutritional standpoint, it's a choice that feels authentic for me. Choosing not to eat animal products helps me reckon with my feelings about the meat, dairy, and egg industries, where a lack of compassion forces animals to lead unthinkably cruel lives. But besides that, this lifestyle has made a huge difference in my day-to-day diet and health, and I think that even if you add only a few more plant-based foods to your regular diet, you'll feel a huge difference too.

Based on countless conversations I've had over the years, I believe many people would like to eat the way I do, at least *some* of the time. They're just unsure how to ask for it or how easy it can be or how good it will taste. I'm always amazed when I join a movie or TV set that's been in production for a while, and the actors and crew haven't already asked for specific food items. They take what they're given, or they bring their own food. It all goes back to supply and demand, doesn't it? We can now find vegan burgers even at Burger King because they know how big the market is for healthy, plant-based options. Yet we still live in a world where many people think the vegan option is simply a bowl of steamed veggies, a dressing-less green salad, or pasta with canned tomato sauce. Having talked with so many people who share that they "tried going vegan" at some point and ended up anemic, fatigued, or just plain hungry, I'm convinced the biggest issue is that their diet was nutritionally imbalanced (and boring). You need to *eat*—and you need to be satisfied and overjoyed with your meals!

Recalibrating how you eat and what food choices you make starts with having the right information. This is the part that many people find intimidating and time-consuming—so let me help rectify that!

How I Became a Vegan—Most of the Time!

Eating healthier can seem like a daunting challenge, especially when you've never thought of yourself as a vegan. It certainly wasn't something I envisioned as a possibility when I was growing up.

My mom will absolutely not mind me saying that she's a terrible cook—it's just not her thing. I can remember her fixing breakfast for me and my brother one morning: eggs cracked into a disposable aluminum foil pan and left in the oven until they burned to a crisp. We all agreed it was best to let Dad do most of the cooking, so when he was at work, I'd usually make my own breakfast and lunch. As a little girl, one of my favorite things to do was help my daddy in the kitchen, and I learned all the basics from him. He never used recipes. We ate meat at least once a day, and the meals weren't fancy, but the food was always fresh and unprocessed—all whole ingredients.

My mom believed that added flavorings weren't healthy, so our meals contained no salt, spices, or sugar. My parents bought an ice cream maker, and we'd have ice cream made from only fruits and cream. Dad would make spaghetti sauce with ground beef, tomatoes, and vegetables. He'd cook it down slowly, and it was delicious, especially when he used that sauce to make the lasagna my brother and I always requested for our birthdays. Although I didn't grow up vegan, this emphasis on whole foods has definitely carried through my entire life.

One day, as I was beginning to cook regularly for my family around age thirteen, I asked my mom why we couldn't have garlic. After all, it's a vegetable, not an additive. She realized it's in the same category as onions, so when I started cooking with garlic, I really went to town with it! I figured out quickly that although the sky's the limit for me when it comes to garlic, not everyone feels the same. Then I discovered and started using other spices, once I'd pointed out they're just made from dried plants.

I stopped eating red meat for good one night when I was fifteen. As I dumped ground beef into a frying pan with the onion, garlic, and mushrooms I had sautéed, I suddenly saw it as exactly what it is—as not that different from my own body materials. I knew then that I'd never want it again, and I never did. It wasn't a health decision; it just resonated for me.

Fast-forward to when I was twenty-four and had completed a cleanse, which I used to do frequently in a (misguided) attempt to quickly lose perceived weight. I was excited to eat my favorite foods again—one of the intense joys of completing any fast. What I was craving most was my favorite turkey loaf from Whole Foods, but as soon as I took it home and unwrapped it, I realized it had become absolutely repulsive to me. Another one of my staples at the time was roasted chicken from Koo Koo Roo. That had become a regular lunch when I worked on *Cybill*; it was a block away from our Studio City set. I'd thought that was relatively healthy since it wasn't processed in the way fast-food "chicken" nuggets are, for example.

Weirdly, what finally stopped me ever wanting poultry again was my newly adopted first dog, Jake. When I was rubbing his puppy belly and the tender area under his front legs where doggies love to be stroked, I suddenly saw that his little legs looked *exactly* like chicken legs. No way would I ever again want to pull apart a roasted chicken and eat it.

After that, most of my meals were 90 percent vegan, but I still ate dairy, eggs, and fish regularly, especially when I went out to eat and ordered pasta with cheese, or sushi, which I loved and ate probably three times a week.

Still, I knew I felt better, physically and from an ethical standpoint, when I didn't eat dairy. If I were having a dinner party, for example, I might splurge on some high-quality cheeses for a cheese board, and I'd often cook fish as a special treat, like Nobu's famous Black Cod with Miso, paired with wasabi mashed potatoes. Long before my dinner parties were 100 percent vegan, I loved making desserts for my guests and impressing them with the fact the treats were vegan. Because the truth is, even if you're not vegan, the last thing anyone needs after a satisfying dinner is heavy cream to sit on top of all that food and clog up your system!

In 2010, I traveled to Spain for a rare "just for fun" trip with one of my dearest friends, Jessika Borsiczky, and we spent ten days eating our way through Barcelona, Girona, and Majorca. And wow—if there is ever a place to have a good piece of fresh-out-of-the-Mediterranean fish while sitting at a beachfront restaurant, I'd say those places are on the list.

One day, Jess and I had paella twice, for lunch and dinner (!), and that night I had the strangest dream: I was chasing an adorable baby turtle through an apartment, trying to spray it with Raid until it died. Although I felt sick about it within the dream, I kept spraying until I could see that the turtle was dead. I woke up with a start, and instantly intuited that the dream was a result of all the small creatures I'd eaten that day.

Later that summer, after a particularly heavy ten days of eating while working on the film *Bending the Rules* in New Orleans, I did a vegan cleanse. If you've ever been to New Orleans, you already know that everywhere you turn there's fried shrimp, butter, cream, and cheese galore—more than plenty for a pescatarian to overindulge in. I came home having had the best time, but my clothes were starting not to fit right anymore, and my skin was breaking out from all the oily foods. I didn't feel healthy either. I wasn't looking to permanently change my lifestyle or my diet; I just wanted a reset. So I went in search of something online and found a three-week supply of herbs to be taken in specific conjunction with each other. The only dietary requirement was sticking to a plant-based, predominantly raw diet.

I also wanted to do a cleanse because I was about to start filming a movie I was excited about in New York City, called *Away from Here*—and I wanted to look and feel great. One of my favorite things about the city was the amazing sushi, so my first night there, after getting situated in my apartment with my dogs, Jake and Maggie, and my cat, Jessie, I ordered takeout. When it arrived, I tore it open and settled in to eat it, but instantly realized I didn't want it. My animals got the fish, and I picked out the avocado and seaweed for myself.

To my surprise, I realized I was *not* craving anything non-vegan. This was truly never my intention. I'd always said, "I could never be vegan because I can't give up sushi" and believed it wholeheartedly! In the morning when I got to work, I told the production crew I was vegan so they could prepare accordingly for meals and snacks on set, but also for any scenes that required me to eat on camera. I realized this was genuinely what my body wanted.

Becoming a Full-Time Vegan

Since I already was leaning toward a plant-based diet by this point, my transition was seamless. I realized then that small changes are key. It took me twenty years between that first step of knowing I didn't want to eat red meat anymore (which was quite a big step at the time, since I'd grown up eating it nearly every day), to becoming 99 percent vegan. So it wasn't as though I needed a total pantry overhaul. It was more the adjustment of keeping my animal-product-free policy when I was on a set or in a restaurant, learning to notice when those ingredients were in a dish, and then asking the chefs to exclude them, coming up with a substitution, or ordering something different. Sometimes I look at it as an adventure to help a provider come up with healthy and tasty snacks or protein options at lunch on set, such as cans of beans or falafel or a package of vegan burgers.

In the decade-plus since that cleanse, there have been a handful of times when I've eaten something that wasn't vegan. In the first few years, I occasionally took a bite of an offered food, like a birthday cake, thinking I'd want to be social or go with the flow, but it really didn't taste good. In Italy eight years ago I decided to order a slice of "real" Italian pizza as a treat, took one bite, and absolutely couldn't eat any more. *I realized that dairy no longer tasted like food to me.* But this was a small change I never could have seen coming—one that I didn't engineer. It just happened.

I'm vegan most of the time, with two rare exceptions: eggs and salmon. Occasional eggs do not seem wrong if (a) I know exactly where they came from and they are genuinely free roaming (e.g., from someone's backyard), and (b) most important, if I'm craving them, which happens once in a blue moon. If you just look at eggs from a nutritional standpoint, they're pretty good for us. However, mass-produced eggs are the result of unfathomable cruelty to chickens, whose entire lives are spent in squalid, cramped, and torturous conditions. (Have you ever driven past an egg factory? The stink is nearly unbearable.)

Not only do we not want to be contributing to that, but that's not a good nutrient source for our bodies. If eggs are something you want to keep in your diet, I strongly encourage you to only buy the ones that are labeled pasture raised (such as Vital Farms). If that's not possible, at least look for the indication that they're vegetarian fed. Why? Because though a truly free-roaming chicken will eat bugs and worms as part of their healthy omnivorous diet, believe it or not, mass-produced eggs come from chickens who are partially fed ground-up waste chicken parts.[4] Also, unless a restaurant specifies where it sources its eggs, you can presume they're mass produced.

Over the years, when I've craved raw salmon, I've taken that as a message from my body, enjoyed the fish, and then I don't crave it again for a long while. We also need to be mindful of the fact that fish absorb all the things polluting our beautiful oceans. We might be better served eating algae or organically farmed seaweed—that's what the protein and omega-3/-6 fatty acids in fish are derived from anyway. Why not go right to the source?

Still, I don't beat myself up on the rare occasions when I think, *You know what would be delicious right now? Some salmon sashimi.* If I told myself, *Okay…but, but, this is the very last time you will* ever *eat salmon! Ever!* I would buy the biggest portion available, gobble it up, and then find myself craving it like crazy because it was forbidden. Most days (most months), I truly do not want to eat any salmon!

This is what I mean when I say: listen to your body. It tells you so much. You can ask yourself what you want to eat, look at or pick up the item in your fridge or pantry, and as strange as I know it may sound, you'll get a feeling (likely in your belly) if you pause for a brief moment to consider the sensation of eating it right then and there.

This free-and-easy attitude toward food is a reflection of how I feel toward most things in my life. I would most definitely put myself proudly into the label-free category in all areas that I can think of.

Weigh the benefits and the risks, in all things, without sacrificing the sanctity of your sanity. If your balance and peace aren't in a sound and sturdy place, what you put into your body will have much less of an impact. My philosophy is that, with the exception of helping you find recipes or a community of like-minded individuals on a platform such as Instagram, labels serve to make people feel worse about themselves, and to make the odds of implementing life changes much harder.

Be *you.* Be your own label.

That's what the concept of small changes is all about: getting to know yourself, your body, your needs—and not changing because you feel obligated or because someone has instructed you to, but because it's the best decision for *you.*

A Slight Digression About Shoes!

I used to have an incredible collection of designer shoes from Prada and Gucci and Chanel, mostly because I played characters who wore those shoes and I got them for free afterward, or they were gifted to me from designers who wanted me to wear them at red carpet events. About seven years ago I came to the realization that it felt wrong to continue to wear leather I already owned, even though I wasn't buying it anymore.

Once I made the decision, I didn't find it hard to follow through; I sold my fancy shoes on eBay, as well as at several vintage stores. I then used the money I made from selling the old shoes to purchase a new vegan shoe (and purse) collection. There are so many incredibly fashionable, well-made, and gorgeous faux leather designers these days (like Kat Mendenhall, especially her hand-stitched vegan cowboy boots! I've been wearing them for over five years and they're still good as new). Another bonus: vegan shoes and purses are (almost always) a whole heck of a lot cheaper than leather ones.

Diets Don't Work—And Why Eating More Plant-Based Foods Will Rid You of the Word "Diet" for Good

You might be thinking, *This all sounds great! What's the first step I can take to adopt this new diet that will change my life?* Actually, diets are the opposite of my philosophy! Diets use words like "cheating" and "bad." As in: "This is bad, therefore I cannot eat it. And if I do eat it, I'm cheating, and that makes me a cheater. And then I feel so bad that I cheated I'll tell myself that I failed, and I'm no good at sticking to anything. So I'm just going to do it again because why bother even trying? I just failed, so that proves I'll never change."

It's a vicious cycle.

I've realized that diets don't work. Over the years my weight has gone up and down, when I'd binge "one last time" before several weeks of drastic calorie restriction or juice fasts with the intention of losing weight quickly before a new job started, only to (predictably) gain that weight back, and then some, after having slowed down my metabolism so much over that time.

Small Changes Are Better Than Any Diet!

I bet you can commit to making a few changes for only two weeks. Or even one week. Or, if that proves challenging, how about *two days* to begin with? It's much easier to make changes when you know they're short-term. As Tal Ronnen said in *The Conscious Cook*, "Forcing a radical change that you won't be able to stick with doesn't make sense. Ease in at a pace and depth that feel comfortable."[5]

During that time, it's important to learn to listen to your body. What makes you feel great, and what makes you feel unwell? At the end of those days or weeks, if you end up thinking, *Okay, I'm going to go back to eating the way I was*, you can choose to do that. No judgment here! But chances are you might start noticing you miss the way you felt when you were making those healthy choices.

Something as tiny as substituting an organic, nondairy creamer (or my homemade pecan-walnut milk, on page 249) in your coffee, instead of heavy cream, can make an impact. The cholesterol you save with that choice can give you room to enjoy it where you may feel it counts more—perhaps a slice of aged cheddar cheese, if that's your special treat. You may find you barely notice the difference in taste in your coffee, or you might enjoy the flavor even more. Or, for you, it may be the exact opposite. You may not want to ever give up a dash of heavy cream in your coffee, but maybe you'll find that cutting butter and cheese out of most of your meals, substituting a few delicious alternatives, will become something you prefer.

These small changes gradually become a part of your routine, and after a while you won't even think about them. That healthy mindset will trickle down into every aspect of your life.

Having grown up with such a restricted diet and rules, I'm convinced that the best way forward is moderation in all things. For example, if you're trying to stick to an all-plant-based policy, you don't have to throw the whole thing out the window as soon as you crave something that isn't on that list. The same goes if you're on an eating plan that may not be vegan, but you're trying to lose weight. If you suddenly have a craving and you eat something that's totally off that plan, you might indulge in an entire pizza. That doesn't mean you have to go back to everything the way it was before. You're still doing great; you just had a night where you temporarily let it go! Enjoy it thoroughly, and please don't waste the diversion by beating yourself up about it, either during or after. There is a time and a place for pizza! (Plus, I can show you how to make even a pizza less of a guilty indulgence—see pages 42 and 55.)

Dealing with Cravings

All of us have our favorite comfort food that we crave more than anything, especially when we're stressed or tired. All of us also have cravings for particular foods, whether sweet, salty, crunchy, or chewy, that we know aren't that healthy for us, but they're dang delicious!

How do you deal with cravings so you can make smart substitutions and try new meals that will help you get to know your body better? Let's start with sugar.

The Sugar Problem

I like sweets, but I don't like refined sugars and what they do to the body.

In order to function, the human body doesn't need the refined sugar that's often added to food, like white table sugar, or more natural sweeteners like honey or maple syrup. But most of us can process the sugars found in fruit, veggies, and other foods quite effectively. (If you have diabetes or other blood sugar issues, even some foods naturally high in fructose may need to be eaten in moderation, or not at all.) Excess sugar is stored in your body and turned into fat, in case you should suddenly experience a need for fuel. Sugar also strains your pancreas, as it struggles to produce the insulin you need to process all of the excess sugars.

According to an article published in *Economics & Human Biology* in January 2020, adult obesity in the US increased from about 15 percent in 1970 to almost 40 percent in 2015. What accounts for this? "The sharp rise in adult obesity after 1990 reflects the delayed effects of added sugar calories consumed among children of the 1970s and 1980s."[6] In other words, the longer people have been eating sugar, the more the effects compound over time. High-fructose corn syrup was unleashed on unsuspecting consumers in the 1970s, and thirty years later, most Americans were eating *sixty pounds* of it every year! Now, sadly, the US Department of Agriculture estimates that the average American eats more than *one hundred pounds* of added sugar each year.[7] This is one of the primary reasons type 2 diabetes has skyrocketed to lethal levels.

Once you're eating less sugar, you'll realize one day that your taste buds have changed. Foods that you once thought of as not particularly sweet will now be overwhelmingly sugary. You might even start preferring the taste of sugar-free, green, or nondairy foods because you feel better, healthier, and lighter after eating them. *Your cravings may change, without you even needing to think about it.*

Fat Is Not the Enemy

Did you know that your brain tissue is made up of 60 percent fat?[8] Well, it is! It needs good fats like essential fatty acids to perform all its duties at optimal levels. And the rest of your body needs fat for energy, to make cells, to protect our organs, and to synthesize certain vitamins.

But not all fats are equal. Healthy fats are mono- and polyunsaturated, derived from plant sources like olives, sunflowers, nuts, and avocados; they help lower the unhealthy cholesterol (LDL) while raising the good kind (HDL). You also need omega-3 essential fatty acids, which lower cholesterol levels as well. Vegans can get them from flaxseeds, soy, and walnuts; they're also abundant in fatty fish like salmon, tuna, and sardines, and you can take a supplement such as cod liver or krill oil, or flax oil. There is also a fantastic vegan algae-derived oil from Sunwarrior that gives you a full balance of omega-3, which pure flax oil does not.

Fats that you want to limit are hydrogenated and trans, which are largely found in heavily processed and fried foods. Although saturated fats were once thought to be part of the problem, in recent years studies indicate it's much more complex than that. Studies, particularly large ones looking at women (the Nurses' Health Study from 1980 to 2010), and men (the Health Professionals Follow-Up Study from 1986 to 2010) have shown that there seems to be a noticeable difference in the way humans respond to saturated fats from animal sources (butter, lard, and meat fats) versus plant-based sources.[9] Cholesterol only comes from animal fats; it isn't found in plants. So perhaps this explains the difference. Even a healthy fat such as olive oil has saturated fat in it. The nondairy cheeses I love also have saturated fats, but in lesser quantities than dairy cheese.

Hydrogenated fats are processed so that liquid oils become solid at room temperature (like Crisco). They can turn into trans fats once your body digests them, even if the label says "no trans fats." You want to minimize your intake of hydrogenated and trans fats, because they can increase LDL cholesterol, clog your arteries, and lead to heart disease, strokes, and weight gain.[10] The good news is that by sticking to a more plant-based menu, you automatically reduce your trans fats intake from processed foods.

Coconut oil is a saturated fat, but its structure isn't the same as saturated fats from animal sources. It has shorter fatty acid chains, so they don't cause LDL levels to rise in the same way, and of course, it's cholesterol free. Virgin coconut oil may also have antioxidant properties and has been shown to potentially raise your good cholesterol, or HDL. Cold-pressed extra-virgin olive oil, grapeseed oil, avocado oil, and others are very healthy for you too—I believe in using different types and not sticking to just one all the time. Although there's been much made of the "smoke point" of olive oil—I avoided cooking anything with it at high heat for a while—it seems that now the jury is out. However, any time you cook with any oil, you're diminishing its health benefits. This is why my preference is to cook with much less of whatever oil I choose and then add raw oil to the dish at the end. You can also taste the flavor of the oil much better that way.

Bottom line: What's most important about fats is that you don't need to see them as the enemy. Plant-sourced fats are necessary for your body to function. Your brain needs them, your skin needs them, and your metabolism needs them.

Managing Cravings

Try drawing up a list of your trigger foods or your favorite unhealthy snacks, and then figure out what might be a better alternative. These are some of my favorite substitutions:

IF YOU'RE CRAVING . . . TRY THIS INSTEAD

Potato chips—Baked potato chips, beet chips, or taro chips made from sweet potatoes and other root veggies. Cassava root chips are high in calories but they're more satisfying, so you need less of them. If you feel the need to scarf a bag of something crunchy and salty, Terra brand chips are a good option. I love their Sweets & Beets made from sweet potatoes and beets.

Candy—Dried, organic, unsweetened mango/apple/banana/coconut are good, or try dates, figs, or a small amount of raisins. Dark chocolate instead of milk chocolate; bittersweet has less sugar but with that same chocolate satisfaction.

Ice cream—Nondairy ice cream, or at least have an organic, minimum-ingredient ice cream instead of one filled with chemicals and heavily processed milk. I love mango, raspberry, or strawberry sorbet with a little coconut cream from a can of coconut milk (chilled in the fridge first) scooped on top. (You can whip the cream with a small hand mixer, but if it's just me, I often don't bother—it's so good as it is!) Fewer calories and fat than a whole bowl of ice cream, and you'll have the satisfaction of eating the same amount. The only thing with sorbet is that it's sometimes higher in sugar content than ice cream. And of course, nondairy or not, ice cream has sugar in it.

Nondairy ice cream bars also help with portion control; Daiya's are extremely delicious and don't leave you with the same insatiable urge to eat the whole box that I remember from when I used to eat Häagen-Dazs chocolate-dipped ice cream bars. I'm also loving NadaMoo! coconut-based organic ice creams. At 550 calories per carton, if you're having one of those days, you can eat the whole thing and not pay the price for it! Also, Van Leeuwen has an oat-based strawberry ice cream that is so good you won't believe it isn't artisan dairy ice cream. And if you aren't in the mood for a commercially bought ice-cream substitute, frozen bananas, blended till creamy in a food processor, are delicious.

Sweetened breakfast cereal—Coconut-sweetened granola such as Purely Elizabeth's. Try giving yourself way more fruit on top than you might ordinarily, too. Fresh berries are my favorite. That way you're satisfying your craving for sugar and getting all the nutrients of the fruit, while also enjoying that good grainy crunch.

White/processed toast—Ezekiel bread made with whole sprouted grains.

Ranch salad dressing—Hummus or guacamole. It's really good mixed with salad! Daiya also makes an amazing ranch dressing. I won't call it health food but if you really need that ranchy flavor, go for it! My favorite creamy salad dressing is perfectly ripe avocado chunks, mashed up into your greens directly and then seasoned. For a more gourmet option, I suggest Tal Ronnen's classic Caesar dressing from his book *The Conscious Cook*. I've made it so many times, I've adapted it into my own version.

Soda—Coconut water. I like Harmless Harvest because they're conscientious about production, and it's organic and unprocessed (unlike most other brands). Or try green juices. I love to use this as a mixer instead of soda/Coke. It might look very green, but it's usually quite sweet as long as it has a bit of apple or pineapple in it. Grapefruit juice, watered down with some iced or sparkling water for a spritzer, is also very satisfying.

Burgers—Beyond Burgers or Impossible Burgers are incredibly delicious, and especially with toppings on them, even die-hard carnivores I've introduced to them are satisfied. There are also excellent bean-based burgers widely available, such as Hilary's, for a less-processed option. If you want to get the most out of them, I'd recommend skipping the bun, which is highly processed and full of emptier calories. Try quinoa, rice, whole grain pasta, or a whole(r) wheat source like bulgur or Ezekiel bread instead; put your burger on a bed of sautéed or raw spinach or other greens, with avocado and all the fixins you like on top; or roll up the burger in large collard leaves.

Pizza—You can buy a premade pizza crust or dough in a store like Trader

Joe's (or make it yourself!), and then veganize it using your favorite sauce, like tomato or my homemade pesto (see page 227), and any veggies you like, topped with melty vegan cheese. (There are also excellent vegan frozen pizzas available, such as Daiya's.)

Rice—Finely chopped raw or lightly steamed broccoli or cauliflower. You won't miss the rice and you'll have room for more of the good stuff! On the grain side, quinoa is also easy to prepare and full of more nutrients (including protein). Additionally, it keeps in the fridge longer than rice does (easily five days!) so you can make it ahead of time and store it.

Eggs—Try Just Egg plant-based scramble, or make a good "cheesy" bean scramble, like the one in my recipes on page 205. A great tofu scramble, found on page 211, can satisfy those cravings, too, as long as you make it so that it doesn't get dry. You can even make an amazing omelet using Just Eggs!

How I Manage My Sweets Cravings

When I'm craving sugar, the first thing I do is drink water. I also sweeten things like nut milk with a few dates and vanilla extract instead of sweeteners, and use low-glycemic sweeteners such as monk fruit or coconut sugar in cooking whenever possible. I also try to turn to a natural fructose source, such as peaches, watermelon, cherries, mango, papaya, or figs. I crave these just as fiercely, if not more so, than I've ever craved a piece of candy. Because they're on the "healthy/should eat" list, I think we forget sometimes how decadent they taste! I also get great satisfaction from making a delicious smoothie, adding these fruits (especially frozen mango, which makes it thick) and boosting it with fresh greens and protein powder. This satisfies my sweet tooth while also giving my body a ton of useful nutrients, and it's a fuel source I'll burn through faster than it can turn to fat. For example, the sweetener in PlantFusion vanilla protein powder is a stevia blend; I don't care for stevia on its own, but when blended in a smoothie, it makes it taste sweeter than the sugar content reflects. This is a great option for those who are accustomed to a sweeter flavor.

More Tips for Dealing with Cravings

Once alternatives like these are a part of your daily routine, you might still experience cravings that will tempt you back into eating foods you know aren't healthy for you. To deal with cravings for food you know you don't *really* want, these tips should help.

Assess What You're Really Craving

Trust me: this technique works to curb cravings. All you have to do is assess what you *feel* like eating vs. what you've eaten that day or that week, and then create a meal that turns into what you're genuinely craving (from a health perspective) instead of what you *thought* you were craving (from a taste perspective).

One recent morning, my breakfast was a salad of organic greens from my garden. It would have been easier (and more breakfasty!) to have a bowl of granola and coconut yogurt with berries, but (1) I did that the last two days; (2) I made an amazing vegan red velvet cake for my friend's birthday the night before and indulged in that and several glasses of wine; and (3) the greens needed to be eaten so they wouldn't go to waste. So I fixed myself a huge bowl of greens, with an entire avocado smeared all over them and a tiny sprinkle of olive oil to bring it all together, along with Himalayan sea salt and some fresh raspberries. It left me completely satiated with the good fats and fruit I was craving, and I also got the goodness of the greens, which I knew my body needed.

Listen to *your* body. If you're not hungry in the morning because you ate more than you needed to the night before, that's okay. You don't always need a hearty breakfast. Just eat something extremely light to get your metabolism kick-started. Some mornings I'm craving fresh juice, so I make a sixteen-ounce veggie juice with ginger and apple and whatever other fresh fruits I might have around—perhaps a bit of pineapple—and I find myself not wanting or needing a different breakfast.

Focus on the good stuff and have fun reconfiguring when you're hungry. Do you think your meal needs to be a little bit of protein atop a whole heap of grains? Or a few tablespoons of protein and fats, filling two slices of bread? What if you took all those yummy fillings and just put them on a plate and ate more of them? A sandwich is merely an invented convenience, after all. When I was writing this I got hungry, so I dumped half a can of beans into a bowl with some fresh-cut parsley that was sitting on my counter, and poured on some Caesar dressing I'd made a few days before. As I ate it, I realized that you probably have the ingredients for a really delicious quick meal or a nourishing snack waiting for you between your pantry and your fridge as well!

For another example, when I was in social isolation during COVID-19, I made a big green smoothie for dinner some nights (see page 204). That hit the spot, especially since I wasn't looking to eat a heavier, fattier meal that would have slowed me down. I want to wake up in the morning filled with energy, not feeling nutritionally imbalanced. Even if I'm thinking I'm wanting or craving something else, I try to look at my recent dietary intake if my body isn't feeling like it's receiving what it needs to run its best.

Another example is spirulina powder. I'm not completely sure why, but as soon as I add it to a glass of water, I feel an instantaneous burst of energy. It might be the concentrated chlorophyll, but whatever it is, I know it's good for me. Spirulina is packed with minerals, so maybe it contains a trace mineral that my body hasn't been absorbing from my food or supplements.

It's Okay to Not Be Vegetarian or Vegan 100 Percent of the Time!

Don't let the occasional craving for dairy or meat completely thwart your desire to be partly—or largely—vegetarian or vegan. If you want to be a vegan but find you just can't give up bacon, then, to quote my favorite vegan chef, Tal Ronnen: be a vegan who eats bacon.[11]

Although some 100-percent-vegans might be infuriated that I occasionally eat salmon and eggs, my conviction is that someone else's judgment is not a reason to not eat the way you feel is right for your own body. I'm a vegan well over 99 percent of the time, so it's easiest for me to say, "I'm vegan." But I'm not trying to pose as something I'm not. You won't "catch" me at a sushi restaurant, guiltily looking around, hoping no one outs me. If conversation allows, I will slip into even the most casual exchange with a stranger that I do eat salmon and eggs on occasion—just for honesty's sake.

The most important thing: make sure your conscience feels right. The choice is *yours and yours alone.* If you know you want to keep a certain meat or dairy product in your diet because it makes you feel good, then it's not worth the unhappiness you'd put yourself through to give it up, nor torturous guilt if you choose to eat it. Strive for moderation, but grant yourself that freedom and joy—the moderation will follow!

When You Eat It, Enjoy It

If you're going out to dinner or find yourself at a special occasion and you want something you normally don't eat, *enjoy it.* Contrary to what you might believe at first glance, based on all the things I *don't* eat, I don't consider myself to be a strict eater. I really like tequila, I probably drink too much caffeine (particularly when I'm filming or recording in a studio), and I'm definitely prone to eating the entire bag of chips if I open it when I'm alone, just like many people I know!

But I've learned to build in small changes that help me feel good about these indulgences, keeping them in the indulgence category and not making them a daily occurrence.

If you have comfort foods you want to cut back on but aren't quite ready to get rid of entirely, eat them. As I mentioned earlier in this chapter, in my experience "diets" don't work because they're usually restrictive, and it's only human nature to not be able to stick to them over time. Never beat yourself up because you had something on your "do not eat" list. Or cut the portion size in half for now, eat it slowly, and savor every morsel.

When You Want Your Caffeine

Coffee contains antioxidants that studies have indicated can help prevent type 2 diabetes, dementia, Parkinson's disease, and abnormal heart rhythms.[12] According to the FDA, most people can ingest 400 milligrams of coffee a day, which is up to four to five cups, without fearing negative effects.[13] But remember, those are eight-ounce cups, not jumbo size! Plus, a cup of black coffee only has about seven calories. It's the stuff that gets added to it that can take your daily dose from healthy to not-so-healthy as quickly as you can say frappuccino.

So I'm not of the opinion that caffeine is bad—only too much of it is. If I can feel my heart palpitating after drinking a little more of it than I need, I know that's one of my body's ways of saying I maxed out. I know people who drink endless cups or pots of it all day, and I can only marvel at them—every body is different. Too much, though, and you can get heartburn, jitters, headaches, anxiety, a racing heart, and insomnia. Some people are far more sensitive to even low levels of caffeine and should cut back. And don't forget that caffeine is also found in many teas, sodas, chocolate, and energy drinks.

I usually start my day with homemade cold-brewed coffee, which has all the caffeine but none of the acidity of hot coffee. Sometimes I'll treat myself to a cappuccino at one of my favorite coffee shops, or I'll make one myself with homemade nut milk. But if I drink more than three coffee beverages, even if I'm working, I'll often start feeling yucky and my energy level begins to dip.

When I'm working a fourteen-hour day, I'll often get my caffeine with a French press full of loose-leaf yerba maté and nurse that during the day (it's equally delicious hot or chilled). Then I don't need coffee at all. Yerba maté is made from a relative of the holly family and is found in South America. It has about the same amount of caffeine per cup as coffee, but it's also loaded with vitamins, antioxidants, and healthful plant compounds called *polyphenols*. Studies have shown that it can reduce heart disease, and the risk of certain cancers, dementia, and diabetes. It can also help with weight management.[14]

Also, when I *think* I need caffeine but know I've had plenty, the best thing I can do is drink sixteen ounces of alkaline, room temperature water. Another wonderfully satisfying drink is golden milk (I love Gaia's). Made from turmeric and mushrooms, you can buy it in powder form at many health food stores, and then add hot water and perhaps a little raw sweetener or nut milk if desired. In addition, there's always fresh or dried herbal teas. If you have fresh herbs in your garden or kitchen, you can put a few sprigs of them in a cup or a French press, pour some hot water in, steep, then squeeze in some lemon and perhaps a bit of a raw sweetener like maple syrup or Manuka honey. (I am a vegan who is fine with mindfully sourced honey in moderation. It feels good in my throat and doesn't have to harm the bees.)

When You Want Something Crunchy

What about that bag of chips I just scarfed down? They were probably made with baked instead of fried non-GMO potatoes, or sweet potatoes, or beet chips. But still. A whole bag of chips?

I do follow the occasional giving-in to that bag of chips with a policy: no matter how much I'm craving them the next day, I won't have them. I don't want to go down that rabbit hole again of eating too much every day. I'll fill myself up with a smoothie or a big salad earlier instead, so when I might start thinking of snack time, I won't be overcome by the urge to eat the same thing as the day before.

When I crave chips and dip, one of my favorite hacks is to substitute the chips for fresh raw vegetables. In addition to broccoli florets and carrots, I'm an even bigger fan of cucumber and zucchini slices. These are great because they fill you up, since they're full of water, and they're mild in flavor, so you can really enjoy whatever tasty dip you've got going. These veggies are great with guacamole or hummus, for example. Because chips are denser, you can much more easily eat up an entire bowl of them and wonder where they vanished to. It would be much harder to eat multiple cucumbers and zucchinis, because you'd be stuffed! Even if you did, they're super low in calories and have nutritional value to boot.

An added bonus for this transplanted southern gal: they are two of the easiest crops to grow in my Nashville backyard farm. There's nothing like picking one fresh off the vine, slicing it up, and eating it as an appetizer with a homemade dip. I'd honestly much rather eat this than chips that are going to fill me up with salt and empty calories. Hmm. I think I'll make some hummus right now and eat it with this fresh cucumber I picked, just sitting here on my counter saying, "Eat me!" in this very tiny cucumber-y voice that only I can hear.

When You Want Some Cheese

Cheese is delicious but it has no fiber, so it's easy to eat a lot of high-calorie pieces without realizing it. A true dairy allergy is rare (and can be life-threatening), but many people have a hard time digesting lactose, the primary sugar in milk. The enzyme lactase is what helps digest the lactose, and for many people, lactase is no longer produced in their bodies after the age of five.[15] This supports what I've always believed, once I started thinking about it: most of us are, in fact, lactose intolerant. Milk from a cow is intended for *baby* cows. Not even for adult cows. Plus, cows have a stomach with four chambers. Their digestive system isn't even the same. The idea that we're drinking mother's milk intended for the infants of a different species . . . it doesn't make sense when you think about it.

If you're lactose intolerant, you'll likely suspect it, as you can have a lot of painful digestive issues from the undigested milk sugars that start to ferment in your gut. That being said, I'm constantly amazed at the number of people I hear say something like, "Ugh! My belly hurts so much. I had ice cream last night. I should have known better!" or "I ate pizza and I couldn't sleep at all afterward. I kept getting up and down with diarrhea," but they don't consider themselves to be lactose intolerant.

Many people also eat dairy thinking that it's a great source of calcium and vitamin D. However, the vitamin D in milk is added, the same as if you take a supplement, and our bodies don't absorb the calcium from animal sources as well as they can absorb it from plant sources.[16] This reminds me of a conversation I had with someone years ago, who was alarmed I was giving up dairy. "What about osteoporosis?" she asked me. "My dad's bones have gotten so brittle, he broke his back bending over to pick something up last year!"

"That's horrible," I replied. "And he's dairy free?"

Pause. Silence.

"Well, no . . ."

Still, I sometimes crave a good, melty cheese. Fortunately, so many delicious nondairy options are available, which certainly wasn't the case as recently as ten years ago. When I'm making pizza, pesto, or anything where I want a "melt," I use Daiya or Violife vegan shreds. I know that at times it's that melt-y sensation I'm craving and not so much the flavor of the cheese. Vegan "cheeses" have no cholesterol, unlike dairy cheese, and they won't back up your digestive system the same way that dairy will either. You can add some nutritional yeast and garlic and/or onion powder for an extra creamy, parmesan vibe to a dish too. In the recipes section, you'll find some of my favorite uses for vegan melts. You can also easily make a Velveeta-esque "cheese" using cashews or even potatoes (see the recipe on page 225).

I've never had an overwhelming hankering for those exceptional "luxury" cheeses, though I've enjoyed them when I wasn't strictly dairy free, so I remember how rich they tasted. Some people I've spoken to don't want to ever give those up as a treat, so if you want to cut most dairy out, perhaps these cheeses could be your exception. Because these have unique flavors and tend to be expensive, you're likely to eat only a small bit at any given time. There are also vegan parmesans that totally do the trick if you want a substitute for dairy parmesan. Violife has a delicious parmesan "brick" that you can shred with a grater. If you like putting a slice of cheese on your burger or in a sandwich, you can try vegan slices. There is even a fantastic line of nut cheese from Miyoko's—creamy and block style, not for melting—that is utterly crave-worthy in salads or on a spread at a dinner party.

∞∞∞∞∞∞∞∞∞∞

I hope you'll leave this chapter feeling empowered to make the healthy changes to your diet that you might have always wanted to try but haven't been sure how to follow through on. A few small and carefully planned substitutions can open up a world of change. It's important to feel as if you can try something new on your own terms, without being beholden to any strict rules that someone else made up about veganism and vegetarianism. I'm excited for you!

CHAPTER 3

Small Changes in Your Kitchen Give You Big Results

If you want something done, what are you waiting for
If you don't have enough, gotta get something more
If you wanna be loved, better start with yourself
If you want something done then do it, do it

—"DO IT"

O nce you've learned the healthy, plant-based substitutions that work for you, it's important to prepare your refrigerator, pantry, and cupboards so that you're not tempted to fall back on old habits. There are many ways to eat healthy without sacrificing your favorite foods. You also don't need to get rid of everything in your pantry, although I take great joy in making this an at-least-once-a-year ritual!

Cleaning out the kitchen is also somewhat of an obsession of mine when I'm a houseguest or renting a house while working on a job. I go to cook something and next thing you know, I'm making a pile of expired items on their kitchen table and tossing condiments from their fridge that are lined with mold. I have a bit of a morbid fascination with how old the stuff is in some people's fridges and cupboards! It's just fine if a spice is a few months past its expiration date. But eight years past? Same with anything like whole grains or dried fruits. Also, if you're anything like me, you can open an ingredient, use it for a specific recipe, and then forget it on the back of a shelf for a few years. It's fun and inspiring to devote a few hours to cleaning out what's no longer good, and salvaging what still is before it isn't any longer.

A Smart, Well-Stocked Pantry

This list contains items I consider essential for any home cook. You can buy them all at once or a little at a time.

Nonperishable Items/Pantry Staples

CANNED GOODS

- Beans: BPA-free canned cannellini, black, garbanzo (chickpeas), pinto
- Coconut cream, coconut milk

CONDIMENTS AND SPICES

- Coconut tamari (like soy sauce, but made with coconut)
- Coconut vinegar (same principle)
- Garlic powder, onion powder, Himalayan sea salt, assorted dried spices (tarragon, cardamom, dill, turmeric, lemon pepper, cumin, chili powder, star anise, saffron, and cinnamon are some of my most frequently used)
- Maple syrup
- Nutritional yeast

- Oils: cold-pressed coconut, grapeseed, extra-virgin olive
- Raw agave and/or maple syrup, raw organic coconut sugar
- Vanilla extract
- Vegetable stock, low sodium

DRINKS

- Milks: nonperishable, nondairy, unsweetened oat, nut, or rice (good to have in case you need some in a pinch, or for a recipe)
- Coffee beans, dark roast, for homemade cold brew
- Herbal teas, yerba maté
- Golden "milk" powder (optional)
- Water: If I'm on the road, the best quality I can find. If I'm gone for a long period of time (away from my home filtration system), a large refillable jug or two is best.

DRY GOODS

- Flour: gluten-free non-GMO (like Bob's Red Mill brand)
- Granola: whole foods–based (such as Purely Elizabeth)
- Pasta: black soybean spaghetti and penne; red lentil penne; mung bean fettucine; whole grain, unrefined pasta (such as brown rice elbows)
- Grains: quinoa, old-fashioned organic oats, long grain rice
- Whole beans and lentils: dry, uncooked (home-cooked beans are healthier than canned and easy to get in the habit of cooking!)
- Dates: whole, unsweetened

NUTS

- Cashews, pecans, pumpkin seeds (pepitas), walnuts
- Nut butter: unprocessed, unsweetened

- Protein powder (such as PlantFusion, unsweetened pea protein, or Four Sigmatic)

- Fruits: dried, unsweetened (mango, apple, banana, and so forth)
- Crunchy snacks: kale chips, beet chips, baked potato chips, taro chips, coconut chips

Other Pantry Tips

Coconut oil is a good one to have on hand, and it can also be substituted in almost any recipe that calls for butter. While many oils (including olive oil) are very good for you when drizzled over completed food or used in recipes where you don't need to heat above 350 degrees, when you heat those oils any higher, some evidence indicates they can break down and lose their nutritional value. Safflower oil is one relatively healthy option—with a very high smoke point—if you want to deep fry something.

Nonwheat flours now come in an amazing variety made of almost everything, including grains/carbs like amaranth, bean, buckwheat, corn, oat, flax meal, potato, quinoa, rice, tapioca, or even vegetables like cauliflower or nuts like almonds. They're ideal for anyone who wants to cut back on their processed wheat consumption or avoid gluten. (If you have a severe gluten allergy, check the label to be sure that it's processed in a dedicated, gluten-free way.)

Quinoa is another grain substitute for rice, and it also works great as a breakfast cereal. It's high in protein and vitamins/minerals and absorbs flavorings well. Try cooking it with coconut milk, vegetable broth, or even fruit juice/compote.

Shopping on a Budget

It might seem impossible to eat healthy *and* stick to a tight budget. I can assure you it's not! One of the easiest ways to keep costs down and to get food that's better for you at the same time is to buy the ingredients and then assemble your meals—rather than buying frozen dinners, for example. (And if you're buying high-quality prepared items from the deli counter at Whole Foods, that's where your grocery bill can really start to become steep.)

Take a family of five that eats fast-food takeout (like burgers or pizza) or packaged food for dinner five times a week. For the same amount of money, it's more than possible to prepare easy, healthy burgers (whether vegetarian or meat-based, premade or from scratch—like my Black Bean Burger on page 232) or pizza.

To help you consider the possibilities, I put together a table comparing fast-food and vegan pizzas. The homemade vegan pizza is actually *cheaper* per slice than either the fast-food or frozen vegan pizzas!

Pizza Cost Comparisons: Pepperoni with Veggies

	Fast-Food Pepperoni Pizza	Frozen Vegan Pizza	Homemade Vegan Pizza
Ingredients	• Standard crust (large) • Pizza sauce • Mozzarella cheese • Pepperoni • *Additional toppings:* • Mushrooms • Red onion • Green bell peppers	• Gluten-free crust • Pizza sauce • Mozzarella shreds • Meatless pepperoni • *Additional organic toppings:* • Mushrooms • Red onion • Green bell peppers	• Pizza dough (16 oz) • Organic marinara • Mozzarella shreds • Meatless pepperoni • *Additional organic toppings:* • Mushrooms • Red onion • Green bell peppers

Total Slices	8	3	4
Total Cost	$18.19 (+ tax, and tip if delivered)	$9.99	$9.04
Cost Per Slice	$2.27	$3.33	$2.26

Here are some of my favorite brands for vegan pizza ingredients, along with where you might find them.

- Frozen vegan pizza: Daiya Gluten-Free Pizza (my favorite is Fire-Roasted Vegetable) at Target
- Vegan pizza dough:
  - Plain Pizza Dough at Trader Joe's
  - Chloe Delectably Vegan Pizza Crusts at Sprouts or online
  - Experiment with making your own crusts by swapping out the wheat flour for cauliflower, rice, or garbanzo bean flour.
- Sauces, both at Trader Joe's
  - Organic Tomato Basil Marinara
  - Kale, Cashew, and Basil Pesto (or make your own pesto with my recipe on page 227!)
- Cheese: Daiya Mozzarella Style Shreds or Violife Just Like Mozzarella, in chain stores and online
- Organic veggie toppings, all at Trader Joe's: mushrooms, onion, peppers, broccoli florets
- Faux meat toppings
  - Pepperoni: Yves Meatless Pepperoni, available in stores and online
  - Sausage: Field Roast Sausages at Whole Foods
  - Bacon: Sweet Earth Benevolent Bacon, available online

Perishable Items

When I have time, I love to go to a local farmers market. Food also tends to be much healthier for you when you buy locally grown items. The fresher your food, the higher its nutrient levels. Not only does buying local cut down on your carbon footprint—and it supports your local farmers—but it means that the produce had a shorter journey to you and often won't have been refrigerated as long, therefore lessening the chances it will never ripen. If you've ever bought still-hard peaches at the grocery store, they were placed in an industrial-size fridge to make them last longer, but they may never ripen after they're removed.

If you can't get to a farmers market, many large stores label their locally grown produce, which will help you choose the freshest items. Here in Nashville, I shop at my local grocery, The Turnip Truck, or Whole Foods or Trader Joe's for organic produce, as well as canned or frozen goods, or to replenish any pantry staples. I can go to Publix or Kroger or any major chain for many items. I've become an expert in what to buy where—for example, tubs of fresh organic basil at Trader Joe's. Bundles of organic, well-priced parsley or cilantro (when they're out of season in my home garden) can most often be found at Whole Foods.

If you buy more fresh produce than you can eat before it goes bad, you can freeze it. You just have to wash and prepare it first (trim it and cut into the size you'll use it in when you cook it or put it in a smoothie). This works well for fresh fruit too. A good rule of thumb: if you can buy it in the frozen section, it can be frozen! Kale, yes. Parsley, no. Cooked sweet potatoes, yes. Raw sweet potatoes, no! And those fresh herbs that are nearing the end of their usability? Cut the ends of their stems and keep them in a jar of water (like a bouquet of flowers) to extend their life. You can also add more of them than you normally would to your smoothies—they're packed with micronutrients and antivirals.

My Perishable Items Shopping List

DAIRY AND MEAT SUBSTITUTES

- Daiya or Violife or other nondairy cheese, shredded
- Miyoko's (or Earth Balance) butter-substitute spread
- Vegan mayonnaise (I like Follow Your Heart soy-free)
- Plant-based cream cheese (Spero makes a delicious line of sunflower-derived ones!)
- Fresh-made milk substitute/creamer (oat, coconut, or nut-based—unless you plan to make your own [recipe on 249])
- If you're wanting to cut back on meat, I recommend some sort of meat substitute (Beyond Burger, Amy's burgers, Gardein "chicken," Field Roast sausage, Smart Ground vegan ground). These are important to keep on hand in case you get a craving—and all can be stored frozen.

FREEZER ITEMS

- Ezekiel bread (pre-sliced; keeps in freezer indefinitely)
- Frozen Daiya or Chloe's pizza—great in a pinch! Gluten-free crusts
- Frozen mango, pineapple, and blueberries (for smoothies)
- Nondairy ice cream and/or sorbet

FRUITS AND VEGETABLES

- Avocados!
- Fresh fruits: blueberries, apples, pears, bananas, mango, papaya, kiwi, tangerines, citrus of all kinds, melon in season
- Garlic, onions
- Ginger root and fresh turmeric, if available
- Green leafy veggies: broccoli, kale, spinach, etc. (frozen is fine, but organic is most important here)

- Herbs: fresh cilantro, parsley, basil (again, try for organic)
- Mushrooms: portobello, shiitake, cremini
- Salad greens: arugula, spinach, mesclun, etc. (organic, if possible!)
- Squash: butternut, acorn, kabocha
- Sweet potatoes, potatoes, beets
- Tomatoes, zucchini, cucumber, celery (organic, if possible, on these too)

OTHER PROTEIN SOURCES

- Hummus
- Tofu: organic, extra-firm, non-GMO
- Just Egg scrambled egg substitute (made from mung beans)

But I Don't Like Vegetables!

When I have people over and serve them some of my cooking, one of the most frequent comments I hear is, "I don't care for <broccoli/spinach/greens, etc.>, but I actually really like this!" Nothing thrills me more. By the same token, in describing this book to those who haven't yet read it, a frequent comment is, "Yes, but my <mother/coworker/friend> doesn't like vegetables, and they won't eat them." And I must admit I've had so many disgusting vegetables served to me in my life. I'm convinced that proper preparation is crucial.

My intention is to illustrate that although you may have never enjoyed veggies before, there are ways to make them taste more delicious and palatable than you could have imagined. Here are the three main ways I do this:

- Hide them—in a smoothie, for example, where their flavor will be overpowered by the sweeter fruits and tastes, like vanilla, in the powders you can add. Use them on something like a pizza, or in a lasagna or pasta you're already fond of.
- Slather them in flavors you love (though preferably not buried under a heap of cholesterol-laden, cream-based dressing such as ranch!). Try them lightly steamed or sautéed with a generous portion of my homemade pesto (page 227) or with your favorite spices and olive oil. Olive oil, salt, garlic powder, and a squeeze of lemon can do wonders, as long as the veggies aren't overdone.
- Dip them in something delicious! You might be amazed that the crunch of a cucumber or zucchini slice in your favorite dip brings that dip's taste to the forefront, more so than a salty chip or cracker. (See my guacamole recipe on page 242, or my hummus recipe on page 240.)

Buy Organic!

These days, you can go into almost any large store in the US and find not just an organic produce section but many other organic items, like dairy and grains. This is a direct result of demand. Ten years ago, organic produce was rarely available, and when it was, products tended to be extremely expensive. Not anymore!

According to the Organic Trade Association, "Organic agriculture, which is governed by strict government standards, requires that products bearing the organic label are produced without the use of toxic and persistent pesticides and synthetic nitrogen fertilizers, antibiotics, synthetic hormones, genetic engineering or other excluded practices, sewage sludge, or irradiation."[1]

Because some crops absorb more harmful chemicals than others (the thinnest-skinned ones, or ones where we eat the skins), you should try to always buy these organic, when possible. The Environmental Working Group is the best source of information about pesticides/herbicides in your food. Their "Dirty Dozen" list for 2021 includes:[2]

- Strawberries
- Spinach
- Kale
- Nectarines

- Apples
- Grapes
- Cherries
- Peaches

- Pears
- Bell and hot peppers
- Celery
- Tomatoes

When shopping for organic produce, I highly recommend examining it a bit more closely than you might conventional produce. Because toxic pesticides aren't used on these foods, you may see more little critters like aphids once in a while. This is especially true on the green leafies, like broccoli and kale. I know from my experience as an amateur farmer that broccoli, in particular, can be hard to grow without chemicals. But usually, if your supermarket's supply of organic broccoli seems to have more bugs than normal that week, another store's will be in the clear.

Don't Cook in Aluminum or Plastic!

When I was growing up, most people didn't know about the potential dangers of cooking in aluminum foil. Our vegetables were steamed in packets of foil; meat was cooked in disposable foil loaf pans; even eggs were baked in foil. But aluminum from cookware or foil can leach into foods, especially acidic ones, so it's best to avoid it whenever possible. Some aluminum cookware, made from scrap metal, also contains toxic levels of the heavy metal cadmium.[3] And when I tested my levels, sure enough, the two that were the highest were aluminum and cadmium. (There are various practitioners around the world who can help you test for heavy metals toxicity, and protocols available online—often including chlorella, cilantro, and a specific combination of amino acids—can help rid you of toxic elements you may have accumulated over the years. And heavy metal toxicity has been linked to all sorts of health complications you don't want, especially as we get older.)

An aluminum cookie sheet is fine for cookies or toasting nuts, especially when lined with parchment paper, but I wouldn't put tomatoes on one; I'd use a stainless-steel or glass pan instead.

Many studies have shown that some of the chemicals used in the manufacture of plastics can also leach into food.[4] The worst offenders are BPA, which is used to make the lining of many metal cans, and phthalates, which make plastics soft. Both are endocrine disruptors, especially on estrogen, which means they can mimic the effects of your own hormones. (This is particularly dangerous for anyone with a hormone-related cancer.)

Plastic containers should never be used to heat up food in the microwave, as that can release chemicals into your food as well. Use Pyrex (without the plastic covers!) or ceramic instead.

And not to be alarmist (balance is everything), but even the cardboard/paper cartons used for things like soups, veggie broth, nonperishable nut milks, and beans, etc. almost always have a plastic lining inside to keep the liquid from soaking through. Aluminum cans, even if labeled BPA-free, have an alternative lining which, depending on the manufacturer, may be nearly as questionable. (Eden Foods, though a bit costlier, is upfront and conscientious with what their linings are made of.) Especially for acidic foods like tomatoes, look for them in glass jars or cartons rather than in metal cans when possible.

The takeaway? Don't panic or stop eating canned or cartoned foods—I certainly haven't!—but try to buy in glass jars when available, and make your own food as much from scratch as you can when it's possible to do so.

My Favorite Tools

Having the right equipment makes meal prep so much easier and quicker. I can't imagine my kitchen without them!

GreenPans

I love GreenPan cookware! They have an amazing nonstick quality, without toxic Teflon, they heat up more quickly than other pans, and they require very little oil. (I also often add a pinch of water to lift food off the pan if it's beginning to stick, rather than pouring on more oil.) These pans cut down on cooking time, cut down on cleanup time, and are reasonably priced and cute to boot. I've gotten so hooked on them, I often bring one on the road with me if I'm going to be away from my kitchen for any length of time. Just don't use any steel utensils in any of the older models as they can get scratched.

Cuisinart Food Processor

I just replaced my small Cuisinart after using it regularly for fifteen years. It didn't even die—it was merely a little cracked around the blade. If you're making hummus, a small batch of pesto, or anything that has a bit of texture to it (like avocado mousse or even salad dressing) this is an excellent choice. I have friends with bullet blenders that also work well for these purposes.

Vitamix Blender

In my opinion, the extra cost of a Vitamix is well worth it. I use mine nearly every day, and I've had it for eight years. Recently, the place at the bottom where the blender meets the blade started to wear, and I called Vitamix customer service to see how I could order a new one. To my astonishment, they replaced it at absolutely no cost! While I know that isn't standard for an eight-year-old device, it makes me feel even better about recommending it. Most importantly, it makes ingredients professional-level smooth better than any other blender I've tried. For making smoothies, soups, and nut milks, you can't beat Vitamix. They're also BPA-free.

Ball Jars

I use these mason jars for almost everything—drinking and serving water, iced coffee, smoothies, and cocktails; storing my nut milk and any liquid surplus; mixing things that just need a good shake, rather than dirtying a blender; canning; and storing dried goods like bulk uncooked beans or my granola (page 209). A couple of them always wind their well-cushioned way into my suitcase if I'm going on a trip. I also highly recommend the screw tops you can buy separately. They're so much easier for daily use than the two-piece canning tops they're sold with.

Shun Knives

There is a fineness to the way these cut and handle that I haven't found in any other kitchen knives. Shun cutlery is sleek and elegant and really holds up to lots of use without being sharpened. And the absolute best part? When they do need sharpening, you can send them back to Kai, the manufacturer, and they will professionally sharpen and touch up your blades for you, completely free of charge except your shipping cost. For life!

Cold Brew Coffee Maker

I make my own cold brew coffee—I've got my next two weeks' batch brewing in the kitchen as I type. (You can find cold brew makers on Amazon, and they pay for themselves quickly as store-bought is expensive.) What's great about this is that making it at home yields a concentrated cold brew extract, which you can use to create hot coffee or the best iced coffee you'll ever have. Even more important, cold brew is much less acidic than hot-brewed coffee; if you suffer from ulcers or acid reflux, this can make a huge difference. (I don't, but I do notice a difference in how my tummy feels when I stick to cold brew instead of hot coffee.)

Cold brew concentrate is, as you've guessed from the title, very concentrated. One ounce of it per cup is all you should need. Fill the cup the rest of the way with hot water, or cold water and ice, and some homemade nut milk if you like. The flavor is intense, and the caffeine hit is perfect. I like to let my brew sit, steeping in the cold water, for twenty-four hours, and fresh grind my beans before making it, so the whole house smells amazing while the process is happening too.

Excalibur Dehydrator

My beloved friend Melissa McBride surprised me by sending me one of these, after I'd had lots of fun using hers as an overnight science experiment, going to town filling it up with every fresh fruit and vegetable she had sitting around. (The pineapple was the best!) If you have room for one in your kitchen, a dehydrator is a fantastic device, especially if you have kids. Prepping the food, looking up the right temperature for it, and making these wonderful trays of dehydrated snacks encourages healthy eating. And it's fun! All you have to do is slice up fruit or veggies, put them on the trays, set the temperature and timer, and store them when they're done. Your whole house will soon smell wonderful.

The Supplements I Take

Since most of us can't consume the amount of raw veggies that we'd eat if we were foraging in the wild all day, as our Neanderthal ancestors may have done, I believe the right supplements can be helpful in maintaining nutrient levels—whether you choose to be vegan or mostly vegan, or just want to be healthier. You may want to try several of these supplements or maybe just one or two. And, like me, you may not need them all every day—depending on what you get plenty of, or may need more of, from your meals.

My own supplementation routine has been informed partially by my own research and partially by consultation with nutritionists, so I encourage you to do a deep dive into this information, and of course, to talk to your own doctor or naturopath before self-diagnosing, especially if you have a known medical condition. Some supplements can also interact with certain prescription drugs. For example, vitamin K is to be used with caution if you're on a blood thinner, and even something as innocuous as grapefruit interacts negatively with certain chemotherapies and other meds.

Once you figure out what works for you, stock up! Having your preferred healthy foods and supplements on hand is a key step to being happy, healthy, and your most authentic self.

Algae/chlorella. My amazing holistic-meets-traditional-medicine vet, Dr. Mark Ingram, recommended The Edge, a powerful raw blue-green algae supplement, for Ernest—and shared that he takes it himself. It's harvested in Klamath Lake, Oregon, and is packed with micronutrients and minerals. I also love an organic chlorella supplement called Recovery Bits. It fills me with energy and is especially fantastic whenever I'm feeling sluggish or tired, or if I've had a long (fun) night!

Calcium. The brand I prefer is Bone Health, from New Chapter. It's made with whole food, so your body can absorb the calcium from plant sources effectively.

Collagen. I recommend a vegan collagen supplement to help with skin, hair, and nails, such as Ora's Aloe Gorgeous, or Your Super's Plant Collagen. Both of these can be added to a smoothie, or just mixed into a little water.

CoQ10 (Coenzyme Q10). This is a powerhouse supplement for your heart and vascular system. I take 100 mg a day.

Floradix iron. Even if you're getting lots of iron from beans, tofu, spinach, and other leafy greens, this is an effective, liquid plant-based iron supplement, so it's easy to take in the morning with breakfast or right before you eat if you're dashing out. I've found it to be more quickly digested than solid iron supplements, and I feel it almost immediately if my iron seems depleted (after a heavy period, for example, or if I haven't been as diligent on my diet). I don't currently take it every day, but I always have it on hand if I sense I need it. Years ago I was anemic, so I always pay attention to my iron levels in my annual bloodwork. It's important to have your iron levels tested regularly even if you have no reason to think you're deficient. Gaia also makes a good, very similar product.

Magnesium before bed. This is crucial for better-quality sleep and so many essential body functions. I sometimes take Oxy-Mag, which is available online from several retailers. It's a specially formulated ozonated magnesium that detoxifies and cleanses the colon; it seems a lot more effective and more gentle than magnesium citrate. Both of these also help tremendously with regularity, if you tend toward constipation. Unless I'm in the need for cleansing, though, my go-to is magnesium glycinate, which I've been told is the form of magnesium my body genetically absorbs best.

Milk thistle and dandelion extract. These help with liver detoxification, particularly if you enjoy alcoholic beverages, but provide liver support even if you don't.

Probiotic. I take a probiotic in the morning, normally Inner-Ēco fermented coconut kefir, or Ora's Trust Your Gut. One bottle lasts for thirty days, or you can take a different probiotic based on your needs. A daily probiotic is invaluable for a healthy digestive system.

Vitamin B12. It's hard to get enough of this nutrient when you're on a plant-based diet. Through genetic testing, which has more specific results than regular bloodwork, it was found that my body doesn't fully absorb methylcobalamin, a form of B12, so an incredible naturopath/nutritionist in LA, Feline Kondula, suggested I use adenosyl/hydroxy B12 instead (readily available online). You may also need supplementation of other B vitamins, or you may want to take a B combo. Pantothenic acid ("panto" means "everywhere") is B5, and I've been taking it for nearly ten years—although you're not likely to specifically be deficient in it, Feline advised me that it helps your hair to not turn gray!

Curcumin (turmeric extract). This is an effective pain reliever; you can take it instead of Advil, and it really works. I also take it daily for its anti-inflammatory, anticarcinogenic effects. (Pain is often caused by inflammation, so it makes sense that curcumin is effective.) I love Gaia, a vegan liquid capsule which, much like the Advil liquid cap (which isn't vegan), seems to get into your system faster. I also like Zyflamend from New Chapter. It's a combo of turmeric and other anti-inflammatories; it's great for inflammation and joints, in lieu of glucosamine sulfate (sulfates are another thing that my specific genetic makeup doesn't absorb well).

Resveratrol. This is a powerful antioxidant and anti-inflammatory.[5] Although the jury is out on exactly *how* beneficial this is (resveratrol is the component in red wine that has been touted for its many health benefits), if you stick to doses under 1,000 mg, it's unlikely to do any harm. (As with any supplementation, check with your doctor to be sure!)

Supplements for Immunity

The purpose of these supplements is to boost your immune system, to stop you from getting sick in the first place. I've been taking Source Naturals' Wellness Formula, a combination of vitamins, minerals, and herbs, for years. Everyone on the set of *Last Holiday* came down with a severe flu/pneumonia that went around, except me, which I attribute to this supplement.

Also, another friend, who was also taking Wellness daily, and I were exposed for hours to another friend who unknowingly had COVID-19 early in the pandemic. She was a day away from becoming symptomatic, and her results from her test the day before hadn't yet come in as positive. Neither of us contracted the virus. Of course, it's impossible to know whether taking Wellness Formula contributed to our immunity, but it certainly didn't hurt! Wellness can be taken daily, if your immune system is especially fragile or when you're more run-down than usual, but in particular when you're around someone who you know is sick.

While you should never solely rely on an over-the-counter supplement instead of seeking medical treatment if you're feeling seriously ill, all of these supplements can help shorten your recovery time. When I've gotten sick with a cold or flu, I'll continue taking these supplements to help lessen the duration of the illness. And best of all, when I wake up feeling like I'm coming down with something (a telltale sore throat, for example), I can say without a doubt that Wellness Formula, when taken in the quantity directed, has stopped my illness in its tracks time and time again.

Also look into these supplements:

- Black Cumin Seed Oil is excellent for your immune system and has a myriad of other potential health benefits. It's strong! Take in small amounts.
- Immune Support from New Chapter contains an array of mushrooms, including reishi and shiitake; it's also rich in beta-glucans, which nourish the immune system. They are adaptogenic, meaning they can provide different support to different bodies, based on specific needs.
- Oil of oregano is immune boosting, especially when you're coming down with something.
- Zinc plus vitamin D3, for everyday immune strength.

My Morning Concoction

Many mornings, I combine two ounces of aloe juice; a tablespoon of Bragg's apple cider vinegar, for its antibiotic and antiviral properties; two teaspoons of elderberry syrup, another immune booster (I prefer Nature's Way Sambucus, as it's naturally sweetened from vegetable glycerin and has a high concentration of bioactive elderberry); and about two ounces of water. I use this to wash down my Trust Your Gut probiotic. This tonic is a great way to get my system going.

How did I come up with it? I was taking all of these things, and it occurred to me one day that maybe adding them together would both save time and taste better. I'm not a big fan of the flavor of apple cider vinegar on its own—and you should always dilute vinegar before drinking any, as it can irritate your throat and destroy your tooth enamel otherwise—but together it all works nicely.

Lately, I've been adding two teaspoons of diatomaceous earth to my concoction (it's full of natural silica, and a friend of mine has been taking it for years for her skin and ligaments, so I thought I'd try for a while), and sometimes I also add a tablespoon of MCT (medium-chain triglycerides) oil for brain function, but not every day.

What to Feed Your Dog and Cat

Dogs are omnivores and therefore, I think, should eat a variety of high-quality proteins. Ernest loves his organic beef, chicken, or wild-caught salmon, as well as sardines, fresh beans of all varieties, and occasionally scrambled eggs. For a couple of years, I made homemade food for Jake and Maggie, my first two canine companions, but I was never sure if it provided the balance of nutrition they needed. However, I've noticed that it's near impossible to find a dog food made with *organic* protein; the vegetable ingredients are organic, but not the rest. I now use Dr. Harvey's Paradigm premix blend as a base for Ernest's food (at the recommendation of our blessing of a vet, Dr. Ingram, along with some other supplements and custom-blended herbal tinctures he makes), and I've turned many of my dog-guardian friends on to it as well. I love it because it contains everything a dog needs for a balanced diet, except for the protein of your choice and the oil (which is essential to a dog, as it is to humans). I do wish it were organic! But it's the best thing I've found that then allows me to feed organic/raw protein sources. The other thing that's great about this is that it allows me to feed Ernest a *variety* of protein sources. This is absolutely healthier than feeding the same thing every day for years, the same as it is for humans.

While some vegans also feed their dogs a vegan diet, this doesn't feel right to me. Their digestive systems and teeth are completely different than ours. Although I don't like buying meat at all, I also know that by making Ernest's food in this way, rather than buying commercially premade dog food, I'm not only giving him a better food source but also creating more demand for that better-raised meat I advocate for. Even though organic, vegetarian/pasture-raised meats and poultry are more expensive than "conventional," the nutritional value is higher, and the lives of those animals are usually better, too. As with humans, good nutrition pays for itself in the long run.

For example, a six-pound bag of Paradigm lasts close to two months for Ernest, who weighs twenty-five pounds. Yes, I have to add protein to it, but pricier and far less nutritious are the multiple cans of moist dog food I'd otherwise need to feed him every day. Plus, dog food has been sitting in aluminum cans (not BPA-free, either) for who knows how long? Kibble is highly processed, so although some kibble is much higher quality compared to others, it's expensive and nowhere near the nutritional value of fresh meats and produce (and lots of it is full of sugar, in the form of starches). You'll also notice that some of the cheapest foods sold for animals don't specify they're human grade, which means the meat is derived from by-products—that is, parts of the animals that were deemed unfit for human consumption. Yuck and yuck.

Cats are carnivores and under no circumstances, no matter your convictions, should they ever be fed a vegetarian diet. It does come in aluminum cans, but my cat, Jessie, thrived on Wellness's turkey and salmon recipe for most of her twenty years and pretty much refused to eat anything else as her regular diet. I want to share, as well, that my friend Robert's amazing dog Mel lived for sixteen years and he ate Purina. So, this all goes back to doing what feels right to you!

CHAPTER 4

"The Beans Do Not Exist": A Guide to Eating Away from Home

Truth is I didn't come tonight to see or be seen
I wanna spill the beans and drink your wine
Download your feed and share your time

—"TALK TO YOU"

I am five feet nine and my weight fluctuates between 130 and 140 pounds.

And the thing is, I eat *so much* food!

People who don't know I'm (nearly) vegan and see me eating on the set are amazed at not only the amount that's on my plate, but also how frequently I eat. I'm always happy to tell them that when you start eating a healthier diet by cutting out processed foods, and when you cut way back on sugar and dairy and meat, you can eat a *lot*.

Then they ask me how long I've been nearly-vegan, why did I make that choice, did I feel like it changed my energy or my health? Followed by, "Is it hard?" The assumption being, of course, that to stick to plant-based foods is tough work. Let me tell you, a piece of okra left too long on the vine in your garden is tough. (You need to pick them before they get bigger than four inches or they're not much use, except as drumsticks to play a rousing solo on the outdoor table, to annoy your friends at your next cookout.) However, being vegan is not tough!

I see proof of this whenever I go to work, as more and more frequently, there are many vegan crew members—including big, burly muscle men. Not to mention all those who start requesting the food I've asked catering to provide for my lunch. By the end of a movie shoot, the vegan options are in such demand the caterer is usually making as many tins of that as of the non-vegan food. My dear friend Adrienne C. Moore is well known from her work on *Orange Is the New Black*, but our characters never interacted, so I'm grateful I got to know her before I joined that show, while we were filming a Jane Austen adaptation called *Modern Persuasion*. She reminded me during one of our frequent virtual happy hours that on our film set, they had to hide the vegan tins the first few weeks or nothing would be left for the vegans. But the obvious solution there was not to hide them—it was to make more.

I think this situation proves that, more and more, although not everyone wishes to be full-time vegan, you don't need to be to enjoy, crave, and be satiated on a much higher percentage plant-based diet than what common perception might be. If the option is there—and if people see those around them eating something clearly delicious that just happens to be healthy and satisfying— they're gonna want it too. (And maybe a smaller portion of meat along with it, if they desire. Meat doesn't have to be the bulk of their plate anymore though.)

With a few small changes, you can maintain your new healthy eating habits outside of your home, regardless of where you live.

Eating Vegan on the Set

Performers, like many freelancers, often don't have fixed schedules. That makes it easier for us to take charge of everything we eat when we're at home. But while filming, I have to adjust to the long hours and night shoots. We frequently start the work week at 5:00 a.m. on a Monday; our workdays are usually twelve-to-fourteen hours long, and by Friday, wrap time is often 4:00 a.m. I'm so used to it by now, like most actors are, because we need to show up for work when our call time says we show up for work. Same for the crew.

Fortunately, after so many years of this kind of scheduling, I thrive on my irregular hours. And, as evidenced by my utter joy at being allowed to stay up until 4:30 a.m. on the set of *Dune* when I was eight—my first night shoot—I think I'm wired that way. It's a happy bonus for me that irregular hours are part of my career and not just something I can experience in my off time. As I type this, I'm eating dinner at 10:00 p.m. (broccoli with homemade pesto, and Gardein "fish" cutlets with a tablespoon of Vegenaise as a dip) and hunkering down to do several hours of writing, which may easily turn into another 3:00 a.m. bedtime, the same as last night. The night before that, I was in bed by 11:00 p.m. and up at 6:30 a.m. Even with my strange hours, it only takes a bit of forethought to maintain my healthy eating habits.

On set, along with our hours being wacky, our eating hours are wacky. I often arrive before sunrise, along with the hair and makeup team, the other actors who need to be ready, and the assistant directors and set PAs (production assistants) who help facilitate the arrivals. I can't eat while my makeup's being applied, because that would be terribly rude to the makeup artist and slow down the process. Depending on when set catering is scheduled to arrive, breakfast may or may not be ready when I get there (usually not!).

Hair is normally the first task—most days I arrive having just washed it, so the stylist will want to blow-dry it, put product in, and set it while it's still damp. If the breakfast hasn't been made ready while I'm getting my hair done, sometimes it's hard to find a moment to eat before work begins. Sometimes all I can have is a smoothie and if so, I'll ask the makeup artist to wait on the lipstick so I can sip till filming starts. If I know it's going to be a day like that, I can try to have some breakfast in the car on my way to the set, or I can eat during a free moment after rehearsal. Sometimes the crew (including catering) is called to arrive at the time when I'm camera ready and due to begin filming, so if I had to wait for catering to get there to have food, I might not have time in my schedule to eat it at that point, and by lunchtime, I'd be famished.

This is why one of the most important small changes you should make, no matter where you work or what your days are like, is simple:

Eat When You're Hungry

Listen to your body and be a mindful eater. Why should you feel compelled to eat only at designated hours or when you have an open window? I gradually started understanding that this notion didn't work for me—and I don't think it works for most people.

If I'm super-hungry because I've been making myself wait until a "normal" time to eat, and I walk by the craft-services table (the on-set equivalent of the coffee cart or break room at work), I'll grab whatever's in front of me to make that hunger go away. I likely wasn't craving whatever I grabbed, but the hunger pains overwhelmed my rational decision-making. This is why you should never go grocery shopping when you're hungry—your stomach will overrule your brain!

Also, when you eat foods full of fiber, like vegetables, combined with a good fat like avocado, you'll be satiated longer. Even a whole-grain, sprouted bread will digest slower and give you a better balance of protein and nutrients. If you know you won't be able to eat for a while—such as during a long meeting or a conference—eat something nourishing to fill you up beforehand. Junk food, simple carbs (like a bagel), or anything laden with sugar might give you an immediate energy burst, but the ensuing blood-sugar crash will make you even hungrier within an hour or so—and especially if you're prone to hypoglycemia or diabetes, you may find yourself getting shaky too. Simple carbs break down more quickly into sugar.

One of my favorite quick things to eat if I'm in a hurry is an avocado. Cut it in half, scoop out the pit, sprinkle each half with some fresh ground salt and pepper to taste—and a squeeze of lemon if you're feeling gourmet—and eat that up. The good fats will keep you going, it has a plethora of essential nutrients, and it tastes so delicious.

If you have a rigid work schedule and can't change your time for meals or a break, don't force yourself to eat if you're not hungry. Don't let your colleagues talk you into eating if you don't feel like it. Have some nonperishable items, like nut butters, handy in case you get hungry later. I also stash dried unsweetened mangos or apples, raw organic nuts, coconut bark, and yes, even a can or carton of beans in my purse or trailer. You can find organic beans of all varieties in cartons at any Whole Foods, as well as other stores. They don't need refrigeration before they're opened, you can tear them open or pierce the carton with a knife, and, as Fat Bastard in *Austin Powers* would tell them, "Get in mah bellay." And if wherever I'm planning to eat has no protein option—like on a set the first few days, before catering has gotten the hang of preparing balanced, plant-based meals—I can give them the carton of beans as a backup plan, to add to whatever else they've got.

On occasion, the timing of your plans won't jibe with your hunger. Let's say you made dinner plans with friends for 8:00 p.m., but you had lunch at noon and then went to the gym after work. You'll likely be ravenous before dinnertime. When I'm in a similar situation, I always eat a healthy real-food snack, like a small salad or some hummus and veggie sticks, before I leave the house. This tides me over so I don't scarf down the entire bread basket before I've even ordered.

Another important and super-easy small change:

Drink Some Water

You might mistake thirst for hunger. Don't forget how important water is. I've forgotten too many times when I've gone out to eat shortly after a workout, and woken up with a headache the next morning. This was because I neglected to replenish my depleted water supply. If you have a glass of wine or a cocktail (or two) with dinner, even if you don't drink near enough to get sauced, that alcoholic liquid goes directly toward dehydrating you if you haven't been mindful to drink a lot of water that day. This dehydration headache can come on regardless of whether you've had any alcohol.

The same goes for rehydrating with a caffeinated beverage after a workout. If you need a pick-me-up, I recommend having at least sixteen ounces of water first. Let that settle, and if you still need caffeine, then go for it.

On sets, if I'm getting nibbly an hour to an hour and a half before lunch, but I'm not famished or having low blood sugar, I'll drink as much water as I can. This usually holds me over until lunch is served. Or, instead of drinking a lot of water, you can make a cup of hot tea and sip it slowly.

In addition, don't be shy about your needs:

Be Clear About What You Need to Eat

Before a shoot, I always set ground rules so I don't show up on day one and have no meal options. For example, if I don't get enough protein, I'll be hungry and start craving sugar or other things that aren't healthy for me. On the first day, if I see that they have a fruit salad and oatmeal available as vegan breakfast options, that won't work for the entire shoot. If it's a job where I'll be on set every day, I send the production manager a grocery list of staples in advance, to be sure catering and craft services have enough to sustain me during those long days. If it's a job where I'm only working a few days here and there, such as the 2020 movie *I Care a Lot* with Rosamund Pike, I wouldn't expect or ask them to go out of their way for my dietary needs. Some movie/TV sets are already extremely vegan friendly, while some aren't. Just like some restaurants. Another option for on-set meals is to go shopping the day prior and bring my lunch—there's always a fridge somewhere.

Since most people don't have catering or a cafeteria at work, you can try the tactic I use when I arrive in a new city and have to grab something reasonably healthy to eat before a long day of wardrobe fittings, script readings, and rehearsals: I do a quick Yelp search for "vegan breakfast," "healthy lunch," etc. The restaurant doesn't have to provide all vegan food, but the results from the search can point you in the right direction. I know I'll find *something*—and I can ask for substitutions. Luckily, these days it's easy to shop at any grocery store—not just Whole Foods—and find quality ingredients and quick, healthy, and satisfying items.

It's not enough to merely ask for a vegan option. On my 2019 Hallmark Christmas movie, *Our Christmas Love Song*, craft services, as is customary, prepared something to tide the crew over until lunch. This is colloquially called a "sub" (stands for "substantial snack")—a salad, sandwich, or maybe some hot chili, timed to arrive exactly halfway between the time breakfast is served at crew call, and six hours later, which is lunchtime according to our union laws.

On day two my sandwich arrived, specially labeled with my name, because by then the craftie gal knew I was vegan. I was chatting with Josh Sabarra, one of the producers visiting the set that day, when she came over and handed me my "special vegan snack." When I opened the plastic wrap around it and saw the sandwich, we were soon belly-laughing so hard that full-on tears streamed down our faces.

As I looked at the sandwich, I said to him, "I think it might be just lettuce and tomato," and tentatively opened it to find exactly that. "They gave you an LT," said Josh, struggling to get the words out through his laughter. And an LT it was indeed: two slices of lettuce and two slices of tomato on a huge, dry bun. (At least the bun was substantial!)

After we finished laughing—hoping no one had overheard because we didn't want to be rude—I found Robin, the gal who had made the sandwich. I let her know that, while I'm not celiac or gluten-free, in the middle of the day I avoid carbs because they put me to sleep, and that vegan protein is a must. We came up with a perfect snack: chickpeas, avocado, and greens. I asked her to chop the greens because it's hard to eat large lettuce leaves in the few minutes I sometimes have between takes, and not get my lipstick everywhere and end up with greens in my teeth. (My makeup artist appreciates this too!)

Sometimes a simple redirect can turn an exasperating experience into an educational one, and you can get what you want with only a little extra effort and knowledge on the part of the people preparing the food. (The same principle applies to eating in restaurants.) After the good laugh Josh and I had, he texted me later in the week to find out if I'd enjoyed any more LTs. It was lovely to be able to tell him that, instead of me just throwing up my hands at the challenges of trying to find nourishing options on set, the experience led to an illuminating chat with the lovely Robin at craft services. She gave me more inventive snacks and told me that she's getting all kinds of ideas for her own snacks too—a perfect small change!—including the high-protein falafel she served me along with lettuce, sliced cherry tomatoes, and hummus. What could be better? So while falafel costs more than a hamburger bun, it prevents me from being extremely hungry and bloated.

My costar, Brendan Hines, who wasn't vegan but is health and fitness conscious, was soon getting the same snack as I did every day, because he knew he'd run better on that too. Then other actors were requesting the same, and soon thereafter, included among the crew's sandwich tray was a pile of vegan "subs" for them too. This has happened on every one of my Hallmark Christmas movies. On my 2020 film, *Christmas Tree Lane*, I had sent a list of suggested shopping items to craftie ahead of time, so they had Beyond Burgers in their fridge for me. The first night I requested one of those, with some sautéed spinach and a few avocado slices. My costar, Andrew Walker, and director Steven Monroe stopped mid-conversation, and I think both their mouths fell open when I opened my to-go container. "Where did you get that?!" they wanted to know—and then they started asking for the same thing as a later-night snack. While neither of them is strictly vegan, the pastrami and turkey rolls that had been passed around earlier weren't what they were craving. It hadn't occurred to them to ask if there was another option.

I think it's also important to note that my food suggestions don't in any way constitute "being difficult." That applies to life in general as well as to life on a set. Whenever I'm number one on a call sheet, I'm working almost every scene. Therefore, it's my responsibility to the production, as well as to myself, to get the nutrition I need to do my best work. It truly doesn't require much more effort, or a higher catering budget.

What I always love seeing is how the eating habits of many others on the set shift after they watch how and what I eat. Especially with the Hallmark Christmas movies I've worked on for nearly a decade. The same production company and crew will often make five films in a row, so the actors change but the crew remains the same.

> Food specificity has become my philosophy anywhere I go. I've learned that I can always find what I want. It's out there. Sometimes you just have to look for it—and ask for it!

After I start working, the crew will tell me, "Wow, the food on this shoot is a whole other ballgame because you've asked for these things." As I mentioned earlier, the caterers have to start setting the vegan food aside because otherwise it will be gone by the time I get there! My vegan meals are so tasty and filling that the crew starts craving their greens too. They don't want to eat a big plate of pasta midday before going back to work, because they'll be tired and dragging. And the caterers realize their assumptions that the crew just wants meat and potatoes, or spaghetti and meatballs, are wrong! (*Titanic* director James Cameron's 2019 documentary, *The Game Changers*, beautifully details the misconceptions we have about animal protein being necessary to build human muscle.)

So if you find yourself in situations at work where meals are provided, speak up whenever possible. Not only will you get the food you want, but your colleagues might start rethinking their meals, too, once they see them. And if you can't speak up, for whatever reason, refer to my suggested shopping list or use these snack ideas, and have them at hand in your desk drawer or bag.

Eat Healthy at Work

You can easily apply many of these suggestions if you work at an office job, or if you work at a job where your mealtime is fixed. Keep healthy snacks at hand, so you can eat something on a break if you're hungry. Stay well hydrated, because thirst is often mistaken for hunger.

An easy solution is to bring your own meals. I love leftovers, because they'll be healthy and delicious, and it saves me the time of having to think about what I'll eat. Besides, leftovers usually taste even better the next day, after all the flavors have been marinating in the fridge overnight. And, of course, leftovers are easy on the budget and prevent waste.

One of my favorite leftovers hacks is to put them, either cold or hot, right on top of some fresh greens. Let's say you had Chinese or Indian food the night before, and you've saved the veggies/protein separate from the rice, which I always do. (Rice doesn't keep as well in the fridge as veggies/protein, anyway, so it's better not to mix them together, even if you're saving the rice.) I recommend bringing your salad greens and leftovers in different containers and storing them in the fridge. Hopefully, there will be a stovetop to heat them on (or a microwave if you want to, although for me, the thought of sending electromagnetic waves through my food feels wrong, so I rarely use one), or just eat them cold. You can then toss the fresh greens with the protein for a fantastic, filling, and healthy lunch.

When I get takeout, I often order more than I need because for the time and energy of choosing off an online menu, as well as the delivery costs (and the fuel used to deliver it to me, the delivery person's time and energy, etc.), you might as well order two meals instead of one. I also love doing this because if I order two things, I increase the odds of getting something I'm truly thrilled with, particularly if I'm in a new city and ordering from a restaurant I don't know. It's more health conscious too, as I've learned from experience that if I get one dish and don't like it, I'm likely to start picking at chips in the minibar or go to bed hungry and wake up craving things I may not need.

My Favorite Snacks When You Just Need Some Chocolate

It can be hard to resist candy or chocolate when it's offered to you at work. I don't eat milk chocolate as it contains dairy, but I do love dark chocolate. If I eat a lot of it, however, I tend to break out. So I save it for an occasional treat, and when I crave something chocolaty, I opt for Hu Chocolate or Alter Eco (dark), which are great because they're small bites. More often, if I'm craving chocolate and don't want to go near a whole bar of it—because I'll probably eat more than I intended—I'll opt instead for a coconut-based ice cream with chocolate bits in it. There's even an avocado-based ice cream on the market now, called Cado—holy deliciousness! Mint chip, anyone? (I didn't say this was *all* about health, after all! But these choices are for times you're craving a little chocolate.)

Mindful vs. Mindless Eating

As I've already shared, the most important component of mindful eating is eating only when you're hungry. But another key component is knowing *what* to eat when you are hungry. It's as important to ask yourself *why* you're hungry as it is to decide what to eat. This can be hard to do when you're having a stressful day at work and want something sugary or crunchy to temporarily make you feel better.

These are the three questions I make myself answer:

What did I eat earlier today? For example, if you had granola for breakfast, you probably don't need carbs, like a piece of whole-grain toast, a rice bowl, or nut crackers as a midday snack, as healthy as they may be. Opt for veggies and hummus, fresh fruit, or a protein source like beans with a little oil, salt, and pepper, or a vegan sausage (I like the Field Roast brand) or Beyond Meat burger wrapped in a collard leaf or atop whatever greens are available.

What am I craving, and is it because I'm missing a set of nutrients or because what I ate earlier today is causing me to crave this? Did I eat a lot of simple carbs (like a bagel with some jelly) that made my blood sugar spike, so now I'm hungry again? Even if I ate healthier, whole carbs, did I have oatmeal for breakfast and a burrito for lunch, and now I'm considering risotto for dinner? (Too many carbs—even if they're good for you some of the time—are unhealthy to have three times a day with minimal veggie consumption.)

How will I feel if I eat what I'm craving? Start noticing the way your system feels after you eat certain meals, as opposed to others. For example, sometimes I crave a delicious thin crust Nothin' But a "V" Thang pizza from Slim & Husky's in Nashville, and if I'm not in town and can't make that happen, I might start checking out pizza places near wherever I am. If they have nondairy cheese and some good-looking veggies on offer, so that I could do a crave-worthy "make your own" pizza, I'll sometimes go for it. (The chains Mellow Mushroom and Two Boots can always be counted on to come through in a pinch, in case you were wondering.) Now, as many of you know, it's pretty hard to order a pizza and not keep munching away on it. (I mean, *er*, so I've heard.) And if there are leftovers, those will likely get eaten the next day because pizza is fantastically delicious cold. (Again, so I've heard!)

But here's the thing: about an hour after eating that pizza—especially if I were to eat the whole crust—I know I'll feel sleepy and be unlikely to get a bunch more work done that night. When stuffed with pizza, I won't feel inspired to write a song. Instead, I'll want to curl up on the couch and watch a good movie and fall into a deep sleep. There's nothing wrong with that sometimes, but I don't like waking up feeling like I'm coming out of a pizza coma more than once in a while. When I'm at home, this is why I'm more likely to make a wheat-free pizza crust (or use the veggie-based Chloe's frozen one) and concoct my own. But in a hotel room or on the road, that's not usually an option.

The trick is to pay close attention to how your body responds to that food source. What I've learned suits me well about vegan pizza (which normally just substitutes nondairy cheese shreds for cheese) is that I feel much less sluggish and congested without the dairy, which makes a big difference for me as a singer and speaker. Before I cut dairy out of my diet, pizza was associated with a real greasy aftertaste in my throat. Now I'm more aware of the wheat flour and, more importantly for me, the yeast. I notice that the joints in my hands feel inflamed after eating pizza, and that's the main reason I don't eat it often. I definitely wouldn't eat it before I was about to play a show!

For another example, did you know that when a certain food consistently causes you to (ahem) pass a whole lot of gas, that means your body isn't handling it well? It's true. Obviously, if you're experiencing this symptom no matter what you eat, there's probably a digestive issue, or perhaps a myriad of tiny microscopic parasites having a little party, unbeknownst to you. (You can try a product like ParaSmart or OneLifeUSA to cleanse your system. After all, it's rude for them to be having a hootenanny and not even invite you.) Often, people don't think twice about this common indication that your body is asking you, politely, to please cut back on that particular food. I bet that now you'll start noticing this constantly! It doesn't mean you have to cut that food out completely, if it's something you love. It just might not be the best food for you, even if it's a "healthy" food. Cauliflower has that effect on me consistently, so after trying for many years to enjoy the cauliflower "steak" that many fancy restaurants offer as the lone vegan entrée, I've finally understood why I could never quite get into it. By the way, cauliflower flour doesn't have this effect on me—only fresh cauli. And I don't care for it anyway. For you, broccoli might have that effect and cauliflower might be better for your system. Just try to start noticing.

Also, how do you feel when you wake up the next morning after different meals? That can tell you a lot too.

After you get used to asking these questions, doing so only takes a second in your mind. Sometimes, you'll answer them and decide to eat what you're craving anyway. But try to consider these questions as often as you can, and before you know it, you'll be choosing differently because you *want* to.

What helps me a lot is to regularly massage my stomach area before I eat. A wonderful healer in LA, Irina Brodsky, advised me to do that, as a way to sort of prepare my body for a meal and set the intention for my stomach to digest it easily. I don't do this every day, but if I'm having a stressful week or a couple of days where I'm grabbing things to eat and not thinking much about it, and especially if I notice my tummy feeling angry with me, I try to be more mindful and take a few minutes for this massage. It really does help. You want to do it in a clockwise motion: start at the lower left, work your way down and then up the right side, kneading deeper in with your knuckles as you make your way around.

Another easy small change is to eat your food more slowly. Some nutritionists say you should chew each bite one hundred times, but that concept doesn't resonate with me because, honestly, who has the time or inclination to do that? Food is meant to be savored and enjoyed, not thought of as a chore!

In addition, I'm sometimes guilty of forgetting to eat. I think it's okay to skip a meal, but being mindful means I know I have to fuel my body.

This is how I shifted in my way of thinking about only eating certain foods at certain meals. I love granola for breakfast, but I don't always need it, especially if I ate a lot of carbs the day before. I think it's good to get some food in your stomach in the morning, but it doesn't have to be a big meal. It can be a few pieces of fruit or greens or a smoothie, which you can put all kinds of vegetables into, and they're portable and easy to drink while you're doing other tasks.

Most of all, don't beat yourself up if you want to indulge once in a while. People bring all kinds of amazing treats to work, and if you want to try something that's not on your usual healthy list, so what? Eat and *enjoy it*. Just eat a bit less the next day. Not being hard on myself for my food choices is one of the most important lessons I've learned.

Making Smart Food Choices When You're Eating Out

I used to think that you could take the girl out of Worcester, Massachusetts, but you couldn't take the Worcester out of the girl. Over time I learned that I could observe, instead of act on, the triggers that remain from those years of only eating in a very specific, restrictive way.

As you read in chapter 1, I grew up in a house where we rarely ate out because we couldn't afford it. We didn't actively think about this as something we were missing. But what was cool (and ahead of their time) about my parents was they put nutrition first. We never went to fast-food restaurants, even though the meals would have been more aligned with our budget than fancier places. Instead, we'd shop at the sole organic store in town and buy whatever farm-fresh things we could get. It was always the best food—not vegetarian, but quality was important.

Later, I realized a rebound effect goes along with a budget-conscious diet: you set foot inside an all-you-can-eat restaurant, and you gorge yourself because you've paid your $9.99, and the buffet is all yours. For me, it was like, *Wait a minute—I can eat all of this? I never used to be allowed to eat this way!* So you end up eating stuff you don't like or keep going long after you're full-to-bursting, just because it's there. The same thing happens with the delicious bread some restaurants bring, or the side order of fries that you may be satiated after half of, but you don't want to let the rest go to waste.

Small changes don't have to be confined to your own kitchen. When eating out, remember that just because a food is there doesn't mean you have to eat it.

Portion Control

As normal portions of food and drinks become supersized, it's hard not to see the big plates and enormous containers as a "regular" size. If you eat whole, minimally processed foods, you can eat a lot more than a "portion"—but try to avoid eating a whole bunch of portions of everything else at the same meal!

If you read labels carefully and see what the serving sizes are, you might be surprised at how small they are, especially foods like cereals, grains, and pasta. Have you ever measured a half-cup of cereal? It barely covers the bottom of the bowl! That's certainly not one of *my* serving sizes.

Although training your eye to know the proper amount of serving sizes for yourself is important, for me, measuring them out is triggering. I *never* measure my portions these days, not only because I don't need to at this point, but also because doing so was part of the beginning of my unhealthy relationship with food when I was a teenager.

For this reason, I'm not a fan of weighing or measuring portions. I'm more in favor of listening to your body and identifying when you're still hungry, or when you're eating because (a) it's there, (b) it's fun to keep eating, (c) you're bored, or (d) you *think* you haven't eaten enough. If you just ate a meal and you know it *should* be enough, but you're tempted to reach for more, why not take a break and see how you feel in half an hour? Then have a glass of water, and if you're still hungry later, go ahead and have something else to eat!

Another thing I love to do when I know I've eaten enough, but for whatever reason I don't want to stop, is to drink a sixteen-ounce glass of water with some supplements. It's best for digestion, though, to not drink water *with* your meal; it's better to have some a while before you eat, and then thirty minutes or so after.

While you can control your portion sizes at home, it's not as easy when you go out to eat, especially with a lot of tempting menu items. The tendency is to order more than you're hungry for because the dish sounds delicious. And this is where my can't-take-the-girl-out-of-Worcester mentality kicks in: I ordered it so I must eat it—if I don't, it's a waste of money.

To combat that, I try to not leave anything on the table. If I'm at a restaurant with a friend and they've ordered meat or fish and not eaten all of it, I never hesitate to ask for a doggie bag and take it home for Ernest, as long as it's not covered in spices. Otherwise it would just go in the trash.

Another way I deal with portion control in my favorite restaurants is to tweak the menu items, when I can. If I order a burrito, I ask for only a small bit of rice inside, as the tortilla gives me all the carbs I need. When I eat out I'm often served too many grains. A restaurant I love in East Nashville, Wild Cow, is one I frequent. Their OG Beans & Greens dish is my jam, and I nearly always order it because it's so satisfying. You can get rice or quinoa, sautéed kale, and pinto beans, topped with this amazing drizzle of garlic aioli. Sometimes it's the perfect amount of kale, but other times they give me more quinoa than I need, so if I order extra kale, there's less room in the bowl for the grains. Because as good as quinoa is for you, it's still a carb.

When you go to a restaurant, ask the server how big the appetizer size is and look around to see what other diners have ordered. Remember, you can always order more. Start small!

Also, I don't look at a menu by category, thinking I can only have an appetizer first, followed by the main course. Look at the menu and then ask yourself: *What do I really want to eat?* That's what you should order, if possible—even if it means asking them to adjust a few things. (For me, if they're offering beans as an appetizer, I'm good to go! I know that even if they don't have another protein source for me, I can get that alongside a couple of sides of vegetables.)

There's another incredible Nashville restaurant, Barcelona, where I usually do have a few pieces of their sourdough bread because it's out-of-this-world delicious, and it's served with an amazing Mediterranean dark-green olive oil that's spicy and thick. I don't eat bread at most restaurants because I'd rather fill up on wholesome food; I prefer to nibble on something like a bowl of olives. I consider the breadbasket a treat and assess whether it's something I really want or I am eating because it's there. For me, the Barcelona bread is the best kind of treat there is.

Ask for Off-Menu Items—If They're Staples, You're Likely to Get Them

Eight years ago, in the tiny Greek fishing village of Amaliapolis, I was having a difficult time finding a vegan option on the menu at the local waterfront restaurant, where my friends and I were having lunch before a wedding we were about to attend. I managed to piece together some ingredients, guessing at what they were in Greek (I'd worked in Greece before), because many Mediterranean ingredients—such as olives, greens, eggplant, and beans—are completely vegan, and I needed to order them separately from the feta cheese or fish. Through my pointing to the menu and communicating as best I could, and with the assistance of the server's minimal English, we were able to put together something I was excited about.

Around five minutes later he returned, clearly needing to tell me something.

After much thought, he said: "The beans . . . do not exist." Our thoroughly charmed table tried not to laugh at this adorableness, I figured something else out, and I had a great lunch—and secretly yearned to bring this ridiculously cute server to the wedding as my date!

When I go out for a meal, I try to eat similarly to the way I eat at home, and most restaurants are happy to oblige. With Mexican cuisine, for example, I usually ask them to skip the cheese or sour cream and see if they have some steamed or sautéed veggies on the side that they could add, besides the usual peppers and onions, which don't provide much nutrition. I also usually ask for my burrito or bowl with no rice—not only because I usually don't want those extra carbs but because many Mexican restaurants cook their rice in chicken stock. In a similar way, if you're ordering soup, inquire as to what kind of stock they use, if you want to limit or eliminate animal products from your diet. Many soups— butternut squash bisque, for example—are also made with chicken stock.

The restaurant business is a tough one, and they want happy customers. Often, the worst question you can ask a server is, "What can you make that's vegan?" which is what my well-meaning friends frequently do when I join them at a non-vegan restaurant of their choosing. (The server will often suggest something like a green salad without dressing, or pasta with plain tomato sauce.) You may find yourself at a restaurant that doesn't appear to offer menu options aligned with your dietary restrictions. Rather than making a fuss, consider the items they do have; with the server's cooperation, you can request a dish using those separate items. I humbly feel I have mastered this art of quickly, instinctively scanning a menu and crafting a much healthier (and delicious) choice out of what they have available—more often than not, the server will return with the newly concocted dish and say, "I never thought to put these things together! I'm going to start having this for my lunch, because it looks amazing!"

Moreover, the world is changing in regard to the quality of vegan offerings at major chains. In 2017, Umami Burger introduced the Impossible Burger, a plant-based patty that contains a scientifically derived molecule, "heme," which is the molecule in a cow's body that turns the grass they eat into protein. I haven't eaten red meat in over thirty years, so I'm not looking for something to remind me of that beef flavor, but my friends who can't imagine going without a thick, juicy burger say the Impossible is the only one that satisfies that unique craving. The Impossible Burger is now available at many US restaurants and can also be ordered frozen in bulk from vegan supplier VEDGEco. And you can find it at a handful of grocery stores too!

Another huge addition to the vegan world is Beyond Burger, which is made from pea, bean, and rice proteins that combine to create a complete protein source exceptionally well-absorbed by the human body. It's soy- and gluten-free as well, and sold in many big grocery stores across the US. In smaller cities, they sell out so fast the stores struggle to keep them on the shelves. In a major development, Burger King, of all places, announced in 2019 that they'd soon offer Impossible Sausage on their breakfast menu. Ditto Jack in the Box. Chipotle has been offering their Sofritas plant-based meat for years. Subway has long had a vegan sub readily available if you knew to ask for it, and they now have plant-based protein options on top of that. Starbucks has an Impossible option for their breakfast sandwich. The days of having to ask, "Do they have vegan options?" are quickly disappearing.

Depending on how strict a vegan you are, you do have to be sure that a fast-food, or any non-vegan, restaurant, is cooking their Impossible or Beyond Burgers on a grill where meat isn't also being cooked, or you may have to ask for them to be cooked in a microwave. (As I've said, microwaves aren't my favorite, though I might use one to soften coconut oil for baking, for example.) The year after Burger King launched the Impossible, some consumers filed lawsuits, because not everyone spotted the fine print on their website and menu stating that the restaurant chain didn't cook the burger on a separate grill.

Here's what I think: a lot of people who go to fast-food restaurants *are not vegan*, so this gives those customers a chance to experience a meat-free burger, and if the Impossible/Beyond becomes popular enough, you can bet it will become standard to prepare it on a dedicated meat-free surface. It's all about supply and demand, and it starts with you, the consumer, asking for what you want, in great enough numbers. It's a wonderful improvement to have this available in almost any city across the US—a big difference from not having any meat-free option at all. Many chains are starting to take baby steps into offering these plant-based substitutes, so I take my hat off and give them a massive salute. (I'm not wearing a hat right now, but I could go put one on and take it off again to make my point.)

Another thing I want to point out is that many restaurants will use cheese or egg in their house-made vegetarian burgers. And that may be fine with you! But if you're looking to avoid extra dairy lurking where you don't expect it, or mass-produced eggs, be sure to ask. I've also noticed that a lot of these in-house burgers are mainly made of rice or other grains, so they aren't necessarily a protein source and will have the same effect as eating other carbs. I share this so you can make informed choices when exploring vegetarian menu options.

Vegan/vegetarian/dairy-free/gluten-free diets are so commonplace now—largely because of the cyclical effect of people demanding it, hence more supply, hence more availability, hence more people adopting those diets on a more regular basis—that all a restaurant needs to do is visit the local grocery store to purchase the ingredients they need.

On the Road Again

One healthy-eating challenge was making smart food choices on my musical tour in spring 2019, when we drove a lot. I mean, a *lot*! My drummer for the tour, Lemuel Hayes, and I rented a Dodge Caravan minivan we named Harold, and the two of us shared the driving to nineteen cities in twenty-six days, starting in Boston and finishing in Seattle. We had a handful of days off in the four weeks, and I had meticulously organized those days by how many hours it would take us to drive to the next city. Because our schedule was so packed, it was even more important for me to find the right kind of food to keep my energy from flagging.

When we landed in Boston, after playing WGBH's *Open Studio* on PBS, I went to Whole Foods and stocked up on nonperishable and semi-nonperishable goods. This being my first long tour, I soon learned that certain things were challenging to keep cold. For example, once I opened my almond milk, it only lasted for a day in the car unrefrigerated. Since nondairy milk options for coffee or granola are no longer hard to find, even in the smallest town, I decided the space in the teeny mini fridge in our hotel rooms was better used to store harder-to-find items. It was easy to head to the nearest Starbucks each day for their biggest size cold brew with a splash of almond milk. Lemuel and I went through a fair amount of those, nursing them throughout the day. I also picked up a few bags of Purely Elizabeth granola, which thankfully is stocked at most Whole Foods (and granola doesn't need refrigeration). Although my preference might be to eat it with some nondairy yogurt or nut milk, I certainly don't have to (first world problem!). I like this granola because it's minimally processed, sweetened with coconut sugar, and packed with nutrients and protein. And, most important, it is addictively good.

I don't like to eat for at least two hours before I sing, because the digestive process causes me to burp—and no one wants to hear that in the microphone. (Okay, maybe somebody does, but that would have to be by special request only!) I do need to eat something for energy, but I don't want anything too heavy. I also don't want a raw salad as that'll fill me up with a lot of mass but only a few calories, and then by the time I'm on stage, I'll be ravenously hungry. So I'll try to get something like a vegan burger without the bun, with half an avocado if at all possible (healthy fats and filling, as well as soothing to any preshow butterflies), and some sautéed greens. When the greens are lightly sautéed you get the benefit of the oil, which is satisfying, and you also get a whole lot more to eat, because the greens lose moisture as they cook. If you order a side of lightly sautéed spinach, you're getting perhaps two cups of raw greens squished down into a little bowl of deliciousness. I always prefer my sautéed greens with garlic and oil, but when I'm about to do a meet and greet, even brushing my teeth won't disguise that garlicky breath, so I avoid that before a show too.

On this tour, because of the sheer volume of cities we were visiting, trying our best to avoid rolling into a new town hours before we had to play—which we did have to do a few times when logistics made it unavoidable—we mostly drove through the wee small hours. That suited me and Lemuel perfectly. We're both night owls, and those venue riders (the list of what the artist for the evening would like stocked for snacks—you know, like those crazy rumors when it's claimed so-and-so will only eat green M&M's and requires bottled water from one particular spring in New Zealand?) came in handy for scarfing down food on our way out of a city. He's a salsa lover; I'm hooked on hummus for the protein and ease of eating; the green room usually had an ice bucket or small fridge, so we often finished our show and then stuffed our faces with raw veggies, hummus, organic chips, and salsa.

What helped the most, once again, was listening to my body. If we hit the road and didn't have enough time to stop somewhere for a late breakfast or early lunch, we'd stop at a market and grab something to go, in addition to our Starbucks. I took advantage of Yelp a lot on this journey. I find it more helpful than searching a vegan app because you can almost always find something delicious and plant-based, even at a restaurant that's not exclusively plant-based.

In the middle of Arizona—having just played Tucson and on our way to New Mexico as we headed to San Diego for a show—we found ourselves on the most challenging stretch for me. The night before, a friend unexpectedly had stopped by my show, and I forgot to eat dinner. Instead I ate a few pieces of leftover rider fruit followed by a few more bourbons than I planned to drink, as I celebrated after the show (knowing I had no performance the next day). When we hit the road the next "morning," I'd slept in until noon. Unfortunately, it wasn't until Lemuel started driving that I realized not only was I profoundly hungover but I also hadn't eaten a proper meal since lunch the previous day. Oops!

I did a Yelp search on my phone while Lemuel powered ahead, and I discovered we were in a dead zone of vegan eats—the first one since the tour began. But I was able to find a tiny café, about two and a half hours down the road, that had vegan wraps. So I drank as much water as I could and listened to The National's *I Am Easy to Find* for our twenty-seventh or so time since it had come out a few days earlier. The café was open until 4:00 p.m., and we rolled up just in time for them to prepare something before closing. Had that not been on our way, I would have instead found a grocery store and bought some avocados, fresh fruit, and maybe a prepared bean salad if they had a deli section.

This vegan wrap reminded me of the time I was at Boston's Logan Airport, returning from filming, and needed something to eat. It was a late flight and very few places were still serving food. The café had the typical kind of wraps, sandwiches, and burgers—all with eggs, meat, and/or cheese. When I tentatively asked if there was an item they were accustomed to adapting for vegans, the server said they didn't do substitutions. I knew this was my only chance of eating before boarding the plane, so coming up with a good option and making a concerted effort to present it as simply as possible was all I could do. Besides, I had nothing to lose.

I did a little sleuthing on the menu, and I asked if it would be possible to get the breakfast burrito without the eggs, sausage, and cheddar cheese, and with extra avocado and extra bean salsa in place of those missing ingredients. She managed to persuade them to make it for me, and it was absolutely perfect.

On the next two pages, have a look at this sample menu and see if you can piece together a plant-based and satisfying meal to order. Then turn the page to see the delicious meal I'd request!

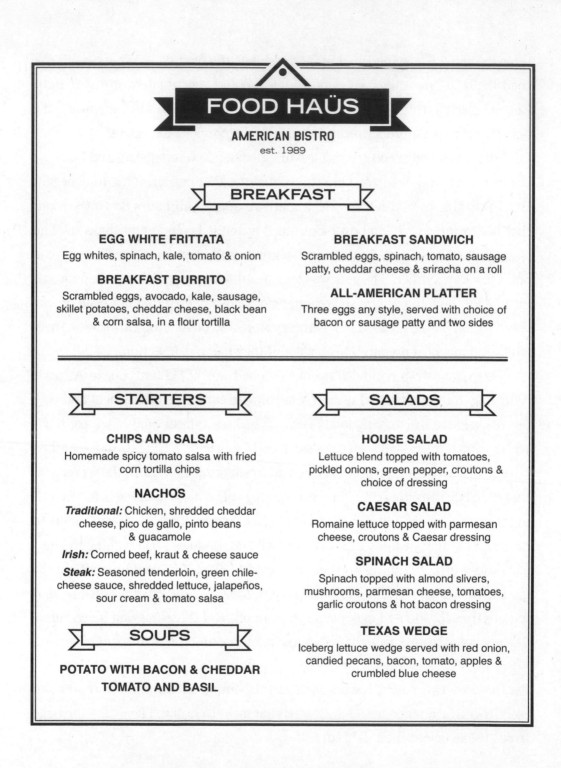

FOOD HAÜS

AMERICAN BISTRO
est. 1989

BREAKFAST

EGG WHITE FRITTATA
Egg whites, spinach, kale, tomato & onion

BREAKFAST BURRITO
Scrambled eggs, avocado, kale, sausage, skillet potatoes, cheddar cheese, black bean & corn salsa, in a flour tortilla

BREAKFAST SANDWICH
Scrambled eggs, spinach, tomato, sausage patty, cheddar cheese & sriracha on a roll

ALL-AMERICAN PLATTER
Three eggs any style, served with choice of bacon or sausage patty and two sides

STARTERS

CHIPS AND SALSA
Homemade spicy tomato salsa with fried corn tortilla chips

NACHOS
Traditional: Chicken, shredded cheddar cheese, pico de gallo, pinto beans & guacamole

Irish: Corned beef, kraut & cheese sauce

Steak: Seasoned tenderloin, green chile-cheese sauce, shredded lettuce, jalapeños, sour cream & tomato salsa

SOUPS

POTATO WITH BACON & CHEDDAR
TOMATO AND BASIL

SALADS

HOUSE SALAD
Lettuce blend topped with tomatoes, pickled onions, green pepper, croutons & choice of dressing

CAESAR SALAD
Romaine lettuce topped with parmesan cheese, croutons & Caesar dressing

SPINACH SALAD
Spinach topped with almond slivers, mushrooms, parmesan cheese, tomatoes, garlic croutons & hot bacon dressing

TEXAS WEDGE
Iceberg lettuce wedge served with red onion, candied pecans, bacon, tomato, apples & crumbled blue cheese

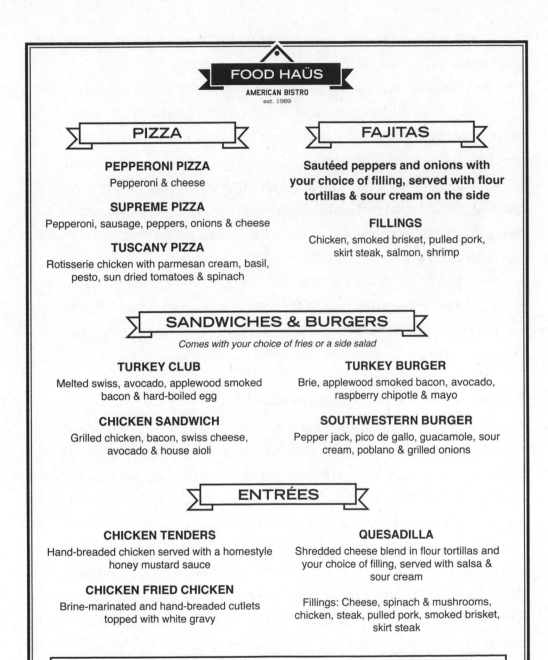

FOOD HAÜS
AMERICAN BISTRO
est. 1989

PIZZA

PEPPERONI PIZZA
Pepperoni & cheese

SUPREME PIZZA
Pepperoni, sausage, peppers, onions & cheese

TUSCANY PIZZA
Rotisserie chicken with parmesan cream, basil, pesto, sun dried tomatoes & spinach

FAJITAS

Sautéed peppers and onions with your choice of filling, served with flour tortillas & sour cream on the side

FILLINGS
Chicken, smoked brisket, pulled pork, skirt steak, salmon, shrimp

SANDWICHES & BURGERS

Comes with your choice of fries or a side salad

TURKEY CLUB
Melted swiss, avocado, applewood smoked bacon & hard-boiled egg

CHICKEN SANDWICH
Grilled chicken, bacon, swiss cheese, avocado & house aioli

TURKEY BURGER
Brie, applewood smoked bacon, avocado, raspberry chipotle & mayo

SOUTHWESTERN BURGER
Pepper jack, pico de gallo, guacamole, sour cream, poblano & grilled onions

ENTRÉES

CHICKEN TENDERS
Hand-breaded chicken served with a homestyle honey mustard sauce

CHICKEN FRIED CHICKEN
Brine-marinated and hand-breaded cutlets topped with white gravy

QUESADILLA
Shredded cheese blend in flour tortillas and your choice of filling, served with salsa & sour cream

Fillings: Cheese, spinach & mushrooms, chicken, steak, pulled pork, smoked brisket, skirt steak

SIDES: Onion rings, Baked potato, Steak fries, Coleslaw, Potato salad

As you can see, the only "vegan" item on the menu as it exists is the chips and tomato salsa. Not nutritious, and not a complete meal.

However, they've got avocado, beans, and corn salsa, and potatoes galore!

So I'd ask for the spinach salad—no bacon dressing and no cheese—and please substitute avocado and add beans and corn salsa. There'd likely be a small upcharge for this request.

I'd also ask for a baked potato with olive oil on the side, or the skillet potatoes cooked in oil, not butter. You could even ask them to add some mushrooms to the skillet potatoes, or serve the baked potato with some sautéed mushrooms on top!

Now, there's no guarantee that the (fictional) Food Haüs would comply. But it's my experience that most of the time, if you ask nicely and explain that you're vegan and searching for something filling to eat, many restaurants are happy to make you happy.

Sometimes You Have to Get Creative!

At the very beginning of shooting the movie *Cowgirls n' Angels*, my friend Frankie Faison and I longed for some nice scotch next to the fireplace at the Residence Inn over a few extremely competitive games of backgammon. We talked about it all day long! So when we finished work for the day, we went out for dinner, and then headed to the liquor store to buy our treat—only to find that in Oklahoma, all the liquor stores closed early. Of course, when we went to the grocery store, they didn't carry liquor—the strongest thing they had was a 2.5 percent alcohol lite beer. Lots of empty calories, low on taste, and definitely not what we craved. We then visited the local bar, which had ample seating outside—but to our dismay, the patio was filled with people smoking, and neither of us felt like experiencing that. It was a perfect spring night, and all we wanted was to be back at the Residence Inn with our backgammon and our scotch.

Luckily, we remembered that in our welcome baskets, production had given us refillable portable water bottles as a memento of Stillwater. Frankie and I promptly returned to the hotel, grabbed our bottles and our per diem (the union-stipulated spending cash allotment for the week, usually fifty to sixty dollars a day), went back to the bar, settled in on the porch, and took turns going inside and ordering two glasses of double shots of Glenfiddich sixteen-year single malt scotch, neat. We'd come out, dump our glasses into the bottles, and after doing this a couple of times, we had plenty of (extremely up-priced!) delectable scotch, depleted our cash per diems, and headed back to the hotel. We got some ice at the ice machine and some glasses—and we were set!

That was our best night of the whole shoot. We stayed up long past when the rest of the cast and crew had come back in, hung out, and gone to bed—and Frankie won back all his per diem and then some on the backgammon board.

For me, the moral of this story isn't about the health benefits of expensive scotch. In a way, however, it almost is. Because in my self-made religion—the rules, or lack thereof, by which I live my life—I figure that if you're genuinely craving something because it's what would make you smile in that moment, and if opportunity and finances allow, you should do it.

If on that night we hadn't found our delectable scotch, sure, we would have more than survived, and we would have had a great night. But my personal life experience has taught me that, on that particular night, I probably would have settled for something else to drink, which I wouldn't have enjoyed as much; in frustration, perhaps I would have then consumed more of it than I'd have preferred. Or I might have stayed at that smoky bar and enjoyed the scotch but had a headache from the secondhand smoke (to which I'm extremely sensitive).

This philosophy leads me to abide by the "everything is okay in moderation" theory, if it brings you great joy. Of course, I don't mean to apply this idea to something you're addicted to or that is a detriment to your life. But I do believe that deep inner joy—and going easy on yourself—leads to a happier, longer life. So just because a book or an influencer or even a friend tells you to cut something entirely from your diet or your practice—or just because that might be what I do in this book!—be mindful, and remember that living a full life, brimming with joy and aliveness, can include all different sorts of things.

PART III

Caring for Your

mind,
spirit,
and
soul

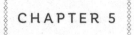

CHAPTER 5

Finding Your Way to a Healthy Inner Life

I'm gonna keep my head up
    like I know where I'm going
I'm gonna look you in the eye
    stare down faith and all the signs that say
nothing's gonna change
    and love anyway

—"LOVE ANYWAY"

For me, good health means much more than how I feel physically. My well-being is dependent on my mental state as well. When you're making changes, you want to be accountable to yourself. You don't want to set goals you can't keep. You also want to be easy on yourself so that you're not relying on the counterproductive "all-or-nothing" philosophy that discourages change rather than facilitating it.

Let's look at the small changes that have contributed to my vibrant inner life. You can sustain this vibrancy even if your outer life is swirling with chaos. And I hope my choices will inspire you to make your own. Seeking to be balanced and grounded, managing life's stresses, and pursuing your passions is incredibly empowering and will lay the groundwork for a healthy life—and set you on the path to becoming your most authentic self.

That Elusive Balance

As you read in chapter 1, my family went to great lengths to ensure we ate a healthy diet, but it was filled with restrictions. Like no chocolate. Or no croissants. Both of which I didn't taste until I was seventeen. When I did, they blew my mind! I remember going to Ralph's Supermarket late at night and buying twelve packs of croissants and hurrying back home to eat every one of them. I couldn't believe how delicious a baked piece of refined flour and butter could be.

This was a new experience for me, but it was wholly unbalanced.

As I grew older, I realized that having draconian rules about practically anything can backfire. Take something as common as television. My mom's list of what we were allowed to watch was very short, and when I was twenty, my friends were astonished to discover that I'd never seen *The Wizard of Oz* (my mother thought it was too scary).

When I first moved to LA, I'd spend hours and hours in front of the TV, watching mindless junk. I didn't yet have words for my addictive, escapist behavior, but the fact that I now *could* put the television on and watch *The Maury Povich Show* in the middle of the day, between auditions, was something I couldn't get enough of.

Eventually, my TV addiction balanced out, as did my food compulsions (which I discuss in chapter 7). I reached the point where I didn't want to spend my free time watching soulless shows, because I was no longer trying to escape from feelings and thoughts I couldn't yet communicate or name. Instead, I wanted to channel those into characters or songs. My enjoyment of movies and TV series transitioned to getting fulfilment from watching deep, profound work from artists who inspire me, or shows that make me cry out loud with laughter.

These days, I'm selective about what I watch, and it's not unusual for weeks to go by without me turning on the TV. Although don't get me wrong—it can be fun to binge-watch a show you love, and go easy on yourself if you feel like watching more than usual for a few days.

No Change Is Too Small

As I've grown and transitioned over the years, my own convictions have shifted—some deepened, some thrown by the wayside. I've learned not only about myself and what's important to me, but also about the world and the beautiful people in it, and I'm happier with and more authentic in the choices I make. They might not be the right choices for everyone, by a long shot. You have to live your own bliss.

Take smoking, for instance. I've never been a smoker. Watching my grandfather die of cancer (likely a direct result of almost a lifetime of smoking cigarettes) ensured that lighting up never held any appeal. My father, the science teacher, also drilled into my brain from a young age that smoking was one of the most destructive things you could do to your body. And he knew how to explain in great detail exactly what that looked like on a molecular level.

The cumulative effect this had on me was that not only did I never smoke, but I wanted to sob when people I loved did. Even with those who smoked only occasionally, I was unable to process it, and my inflexible rejection of the habit helped destroy several romantic relationships when I was much younger. The import I placed on whether someone had one or two cigarettes once in a while could outweigh all else that was good and make me not want to be with them anymore. (Talk about not finding a healthy balance!)

I have other friends whose parental disapproval of smoking actually *caused* them to pick up the habit, in rebellion. It was something they did not because they loved it but because they wanted to escape—and then they became hooked. As with my experiences that I've already shared, strict rules often backfire.

If you care about someone else's well-being, one of the absolute worst ways to effect change is to lecture, however well-meaning. Thinking that "because *I'm* not a smoker, no one else should be either" is dangerously unbalanced. Who am I to say? What if someone loves smoking so much they're willing to accept the risks? It's not my place to judge.

I've had this very conversation with the two people closest to me in my life who have been lifelong smokers, when they brought up their habit as something they *know* they shouldn't be doing. "It's your life," I told them. "Only you know how you want to live it." And I meant it.

To my unbridled joy, a few months later, they both shared with me that they'd started cutting back. I don't know if this was a coincidence—I'm certainly not taking one shred of credit for their decisions, or whether they prove to be long-term ones—but you never know how a kind, balanced comment can resonate with the people who most need to hear it.

Trust Yourself and What You Believe In

While striving to bring more balance into your life—juggling the demands of work, family, friends, and everything going on in the world—you'll drive yourself crazy if you try to find the "right" way to do anything. There will always be a million studies, online commentators, and conspiracy theories to undermine your confidence, even if you know in your heart that something's the best way for you.

All we can control is how we, ourselves, behave. How we treat others. How we try to be a light for good as we live our lives. If we live in fear, that accomplishes nothing. I believe one key to finding that elusive balance is to listen, to form your own opinions, and to not use labels. When you label, it's easy to fall into a "I am this, and you are that, and if you don't agree with me, we're enemies" kind of stance.

Make the choices that feel right in your heart. Be flexible enough to shift gears if your initial path isn't working for you. If we're all willing to do that and accept that in others—even those with whom we disagree—we'd all be working toward a common goal and honoring our existence and that of all other beings on this beautiful, fragile planet of ours. We stand a much better chance as a society, and as a world, if we start making small changes where we can.

I often think about this when I'm in a grocery store and walk by the meat section. Some people think about vegan meat substitutes the way I think about meat: that is, they find the idea of eating them to be repulsive. And I understand that if *everyone* on the planet instantly ended their meat consumption, without a transition period, a lot of meat farmers would be facing financial ruin, with no time to shift to a different livelihood. However, it's been happening gradually, and now there are many inspiring stories of lifelong cattle or chicken farmers moving toward plant-based crops and performing better financially.[1]

During the COVID-19 pandemic, many meat-packing plants became hot-beds for spreading the virus nationwide. I will burst into tears right now if I start telling you about the hundreds of thousands of animal lives intended for human consumption that were killed and disposed of—without their precious lives and bodies even being used as food—because there was no way to process them during that time.[2]

Conversely, if you eat Beyond or Impossible Burgers twice a day, every day, that's also imbalanced. Variety is essential for maintaining a healthy diet. If you want to switch to almond milk because you know cow's milk isn't good for you or the planet, but then you read about how water-intensive growing almond crops is, this might make you worry that trying to be sustainable can backfire. (Oat milk is an excellent alternative.[3]) Same goes for soy being overplanted to the extent that some nutritionists say it's nearly all genetically modified, even if the label says it's organic (which means it's also supposed to be non-GMO).[4] The point is, you can truly drive yourself crazy. Please don't!

Exploring the issues will help you balance the pros and cons and make informed decisions about what you want and need. Instead of giving up because you think your small changes don't matter, start with something easy to do.

For instance, when shopping, faced with a choice between plastic and glass containers, always choose glass if you can. Use compostable bags for your trash instead of the plastic ones, which are estimated to take up to a thousand years to break down—even though the compostable bags sometimes aren't as strong. Let's increase the demand, and the quality and strength will improve. (The JTSC brand, which you can order online, works best of the ones I've tried.) Bags labeled only biodegradable, but not compostable, will equally take forever to biodegrade if they're being used for trash. If they're put in a landfill, they won't get the sunlight they'd need to biodegrade. Or eat more organic and whole foods, and perhaps start substituting high-quality plant-based proteins for some of the meat. See how you feel about these kinds of changes—see if they're right for you.

For relationships, recognize that someone else's ego or insecurities are usually at the core of difficult personalities, and people acting out are often doing so because something in them is deeply unhappy. There've been times even in recent years when I've come home from the set and felt as though I didn't handle problem situations with as much peace as I should have. But to my relief and surprise, I've heard from others who were present that they admired how I kept my cool and addressed the situation directly, but without losing my temper. This tells me I'm progressing. I may not feel that way inside, but I realize from experience that the more connected I remain to my truth, the more peace I can maintain and reflect—thereby creating a more peaceful experience for those with whom I interact.

I'm an actor who's never studied acting, and I believe there's no right or wrong way. I've worked with many actors who swear by one technique or another and who continue to study, and I've worked with many who are also untrained. I've learned myriad lessons in terms of how to conduct myself at work, especially around trying to strike the right balance between being easygoing, and protecting my process—while never, never making it about my ego. Because I'm an instinctive actor, I need to be in a place of letting my interpretation of the character flow out, and then work from there with the director on what that interpretation should be, to best serve the project. I think I work well with most people, but some directors tend to focus on what the work *looks* like and provide guidance from that viewpoint, rather than direct from emotional motivation.

Here's one example: I was filming a scene where my character is in the depths of despair, having just lost her husband as an unintended result of her own actions. (It was a medieval fable.) As she prepares to send her love off on a funeral pyre, I was crying genuine tears that I'd worked myself up into. The director came over after our first take and, without a moment's hesitation, said, "It looks shitty when you sniffle like that. Can you not cry so much? Maybe a tear or two...," as he gestured to the eye he wished said tear to roll from. In a nanosecond, I was out of the mood, confused, and hyperaware of what my face was doing. The actor popped up from his corpse-acting on the pyre and started yelling at him, in their native German, "You can't say that to an actor! Have you lost your mind?" It was pretty funny even at the time! Now, I do know what the director wanted, and I'm sure he was right, but this direction was visually based. A motivation-based direction would be, "Let's try a take where your character has already cried all her tears, and now she's resigned to saying goodbye."

From the get-go, I can quickly identify when directors are inclined to over-direct me. For me, this isn't conducive to getting what they're hoping for. When that happens, I need to stand up for what allows me to provide the best perfor-mance, because I finally understand that's part of what I've been hired to do.

In any relationship—professional or otherwise—it's important to calmly let a collaborator know if they're providing you instruction or communica-tion that's undermining your ability to do your best work. But speaking up for myself hasn't always been easy. Although I don't hesitate now to address something when I think it will help, I still need to quell a shaky feeling when I do so. Plus, if the director doesn't understand where I'm coming from, when I go home that night, I can slip into fearing I've come off as a diva.

I often discuss this topic with my female friends. Even in this day and age, a lot of women I know balk at saying something isn't working for them, out of a deep-seated fear that we'll be seen as needy or emotional or ruthlessly ambitious. As though any of those things are bad qualities! Most men I know don't share this concern. The truth is: speaking straightforwardly—when you take fear *out of* the equation—is the best chance you have to convey your message and create a drama-free work environment. The fear itself causes you to approach someone with frustration—or to wait until the situation has reached a boiling point, prompting you to react in a more heated way than you intended to. When you come from a place of productivity, rather than a place of ego, you don't have to fear that directness. A real strength comes from being unafraid to tell someone that a different way of communicating might be helpful. In other words, you're striving to balance your own needs (being told what's expected of you in an effective way) with someone else's long-standing patterns of communication that they're probably unaware of.

Not everybody is going to be your tribe member. Sometimes you have jobs with people who don't speak the same language you do, figuratively speaking, but you have to make it work anyway. The constant balance is assessing whether it's worth bringing up a problem or riding it out. It's unproductive and harmful to your soul to internalize any sort of professional criticism and take it to a personal place within yourself.

Often, the greatest lesson you can take away from someone who's disappointed you is not to get angry, but to allow yourself to consider what that person must be going through to cause them to express themselves in a hurtful way. Try to take these as learning experiences, rather than proof that all people are alike and will let you down. (Although even the most loyal people in your life will at some point, and it's not the end of the world—another important thing to remember.) Push away the upset and don't blame yourself. People often only lash out in extreme anger when they know they've done something they shouldn't have or that they feel guilty about. Realizing this can help so much when someone snaps at you, or seems to make an accusation out of the blue.

You are your own ambassador. You don't have to preach to change the world. Lead by example, and watch what happens!

Interacting with people of all sorts is a reality of life. What you have ultimate control over is *your* reaction. As you start to feel comfortable with your own power, you'll become clearer about which situations are unacceptable to you, requiring you to look at removing yourself from them—and which ones need you to adjust your handling of them.

Finding Balance When Your Schedule Is Unpredictable

It's not always easy to balance professional and personal commitments.

Sometimes I feel like my life is getting out of control, especially with how unstructured the work is for my profession(s). When I'm working on a TV series or film, my shooting schedule is inflexible and the hours are insane, sometimes with sixteen- or seventeen-hour workdays. When the weekend comes, I just need to sleep. Then, there are times I have a few months off, and, because I'm such a free-flowing person, suddenly my hours are all over the place. Needing to rely solely on myself to push my life forward has taught me a lot about balance, and also motivation.

Conversely, if you have a family and that kind of constant demand on your time and energy, you may not lack daily structure, but you may feel similarly overwhelmed by a stream of days in which you wake up and you're off to the races, and before you know it, the day's over, and you have to start all over again.

These are my favorite simple tips for managing an unpredictable schedule:

- Make lists. Writing things down not only helps you remember them but crossing off items as they're done is extremely satisfying—and a reminder that you're setting goals and meeting them.
- Stock your pantry and fridge with staples, so you can eat well even if you end up with less time than you expected for meal preparation.
- Always find some time to exercise and/or meditate. Even if it's only for a few minutes each day, this will help you feel centered and in control. (In the next chapter, you'll find lots of tips on this topic.)
- Keep a small bag filled with your travel-size essentials so that you can throw it in your car or whatever bag you have with you. I always have the following handy: lip balm, a small fragrance oil, a prescription-bottle size of Wellness Formula, a thermos of water, and a sample-size sunscreen.

- If you have to cancel plans with someone at the last minute, schedule another plan at the same time, and offer to buy the first round of drinks or appetizers, or to pick them up, etc. This practice can keep you holding to your plans more often than not. And by being someone who shows up when you say you will, you'll attract that in those around you. (Having lived in LA for so long, I know how easy it is to fall into a culture of canceling two hours prior. This should be the exception and not the norm, I say.)
- Create a bedtime routine that gives you a sense of continuity wherever you may be, and regardless of whatever time you go to bed from night to night. If you have trouble sleeping due to your schedule or if outside noises wake you easily, earplugs, a sleep mask, aromatherapy oils, or a relaxing white noise or peaceful sounds app can help you relax.

Weaning Yourself Off Social Media

Social media can give you either a sense of well-being or a sense of queasiness, based on what you're absorbing there. Whether you're using your socials to keep up with your family, promote your business, get your news, or all of the above, be mindful of how it affects your mood and energy. I love how we can connect with others through social media, and I greatly appreciate the importance of using it to disseminate information, or for artists to keep people up to date on new projects—I discover lots of my favorite new music, movies, etc. that way. And while I love social media for finding tribe members in a large, collective sense, I know there's way too much negativity as well. Again, we need to take care of ourselves first and foremost; only then can we take care of others.

If you're getting embroiled in personal and heated debates every time you open up socials, that doesn't help with anything. I'm not in favor of avoiding all people with whom I disagree, and if someone is kind and has a well-thought-out point of view that differs from mine, I'm happy to hear it and exchange thoughts.

Name-calling, or continuously attempting to force your opinion on someone for the sake of goading them, is never helpful. The less we engage in these kinds of behaviors, the better off we all are.

Given the pace of modern life and how much information is blessedly available at our fingertips, it's easy to find yourself absentmindedly thumbing through social media feeds as time ticks away. This can happen when you're exhausted and you've already accomplished everything constructive you planned to do that day—or when you're in the middle of work and something on social media feeds distracts you and hooks you in. I think these sites reel you by almost making you feel as if all the accounts you follow are unread messages, and you can't put down your phone till you've seen them all. Except you'll never be at the end—there's always more. Suddenly, half an hour has gone by. When this happens to me, I know I need to set limits for myself.

Whenever I feel the pull to mindlessly scroll or zone out in front of the TV, I've taught myself a few easy tricks. Routines are immensely helpful. The more you can stick to certain ones, such as at bedtime, the more you'll find yourself looking forward to them. If you feel you're settling into a place where you're about to burn through time beyond unwinding or taking a break, reach for one of the routines in chapter 6.

For example, on the day in October 2020 when I'd planned to spend my afternoon finishing the first draft of this chapter, I started with an early morning hike with a friend. The stress of doing so with masks on—and dodging the majority of hikers who weren't wearing them—as well as wondering when I'd be able to safely see my parents again, and dealing with a mounting to-do list of deadlines, added up to me feeling overwhelmed. Yet the more I tried to work, the less creative or productive I felt. I ended up ticking off some of those to-do-list items, and then, realizing it was Sunday, I decided to order takeout, watch a movie, and go to bed early. I stuck to my bedtime routine, eager to get into it early and finish with my gratitude journal.

What ended up happening surprised me. By giving myself permission to take the day off, I ended up with a second wind after my shower, and instead of going to bed, I finished this chapter! Even though I got less sleep, I slept sounder and more peacefully knowing that not only did I get my well-earned rest, but I also completed my original goal.

Discovering Your Resilience When Stress Becomes Overwhelming

I think of resilience as the art of reinventing yourself, over and over if need be—taking the lessons that come your way, the joyful ones and the painful ones, and letting them lead you to the best version of you that you can be at that moment. Resilience is the art of not letting a bad day or a tough break *break* you, but letting it absorb into your membrane and reshape your very core, so you can rise up into the tomorrow you were born to live. Resilience is the definition of what we all need to survive and to thrive. And if ever a year taught us this, it was 2020.

The gift of being an actor has given me the unique experience of learning about resilience through many of the characters I've played. Two that come to mind immediately are Wendy Crowe in *Justified*, and Zelda in *Orange Is the New Black*. Wendy starts season five in a position she has seemingly been in for a while: caught between loyalty to her family of hustlers—each one comically dumber than the last—and her assertion to law enforcement that she's earning an honest living and doing her best to separate herself from her family's crooked ways. As the season progresses, it becomes clear she can't choose both lives any longer, and she needs to stand up for herself in ways she hasn't before, moving through being utterly beaten down to finding the strength to rise up for good. She finds herself strong because she doesn't have a choice.

Zelda was confident and empathic, making a great living for herself and enjoying the luxuries that life affords her, while remaining spontaneous and totally at ease wherever she was. I loved her genuine swagger, the owning of all she had to offer. She was also enviably confident in her romantic life—having just gotten out of a long-term marriage, I admired her go-big-or-go-home focus in pursuing Piper and making her interest unmistakable. But I also loved that she's not one to sit around pining when the object of her affection chooses another. She has way too high an opinion of herself for that! While I was playing her, I often found myself thinking, *What would Zelda do?* in my real life, and I still summon her in my mind when I need an extra boost of inner light.

Similarly, I think most of us can recall moments in which we've been especially proud of ourselves, as well as moments we've observed in people we admire. The definition of personal resilience is different for each of us, and we can draw on these examples when needed.

Many of us will also need to "play a role" from time to time in our lives, at work or in personal situations, which isn't the same as lying or being inauthentic. We all sometimes need to lead with an external reaction that we only wish could reflect our unfiltered internal reaction! However, we can let those experiences illuminate our inner strength and resilience. After all, if you face a challenging situation and have to think fast, keep a cool head, and quickly suss out the right things to say or do, even if you're reeling inside, that is all *you*. Then, when the pressure isn't on, you can think back to that occasion and remember that you're a superhero!

When you think about it, there's something strange about one or several human beings standing on a platform and being the center of attention while a crowd of other human beings watch them! Whether you're giving a speech, playing a song, or leading a board meeting, it can be unsettling to experience the sensation that all eyes are on you. Leveling that physical platform in your own head can help center you back to *why* you're up on that stage: to connect with others.

Same goes if you've been hired for a position that sometimes makes you wonder if you're qualified enough or the right fit. It can be a fine line between humility and forgetting your own strength. You were definitely hired to stand in your own power and light! You do everyone around you a favor when you carry yourself as though you have a unique purpose, whatever the scenario—because I can promise you, you do. Look back at all the stressful situations you've already overcome and realize that your resilience is always there to draw upon when you need it the most.

Asking for Emotional Support

I am lucky that friends, family, and emotional support are now an integral part of my life to help me keep things in perspective when stress threatens to get out of hand.

I'm also fortunate to have found such an amazing community of women in Nashville. One major reason that living here feels so much like home to me is my core group of trusted friends. Some of the most extraordinary women I've ever met live less than twenty minutes away, and knowing we all have each other's back and love each other like chosen family through thick and thin is a great comfort.

When one of us is ill or hospitalized, the others rally to help; we always come to each other's aid when we need dog-sitting or help with anything at all—a commitment only the isolation of a pandemic like COVID-19 could shake. One member of this beloved group contracted this virus, and as many readers sadly know, nothing is more painful than not being able to be there for a loved one as they struggle with this horribly contagious disease.

For instance, on the day the moving truck pulled up from LA with all my belongings, it immediately started downpouring with one of our famous southern spring storms. The movers were on the clock and couldn't stop the move-in process. In a panic, seeing these boxes come in soaking wet and water pooling all over my newly varnished floors and freshly painted walls, I texted my dear friends Fran, Paula, and Vanessa: "SOS—please bring towels if any of you are around." All of my towels were still packed in one of the hundreds of boxes! Within ten minutes, all three of them showed up with piles of towels. They stayed until 12:30 a.m., helping me unpack my soggy boxes and putting away all my kitchen supplies. I woke up the next morning already half-unpacked, feeling unspeakably grateful. That's the sort of chosen family you can't find just anywhere.

Reaching out and asking for help is something we should all do when needed. You may find that reaching out to people you trust encourages them to feel safe to do the same. And it's nothing to feel embarrassed about if they don't get back to you right away, or if you pour your heart out and they're not in a place where they feel comfortable doing the same thing.

This has been a long time coming for me, but I've felt more peaceful since I started opening up whenever I want to, with whomever I feel compelled to— but with no expectation of how the other person needs to reply. If they don't reciprocate . . . well, as long as that wasn't your end goal in reaching out, then it doesn't matter, does it?

Some of us tend to take everything so very personally. I've found it's easier and healthier for me to never pin my happiness on anyone else, even a partner. It comes back to self-sufficiency, but within that, the strength to ask for help. If you don't find it from one person you reach out to, reach out to another—or five more. You'll find that you're not alone. There is strength in acknowledging you need affirmation sometimes—and figuring out who your go-to people are whom you can count on.

There is also much to be said about finding an area to live that resonates with you. You can feel a misalignment within if your location isn't right. My day-to-day in LA didn't usually include spending quality time with even the people I was closest to. The spread-out structure of LA, coupled with its traffic gridlock, hindered making plans. My days were often spent alone in my beautiful, isolated house with amazing canyon views. It was lovely, but I craved community.

By the same token, sometimes it's not the city but the circle you've built that's not quite resonating with you, and you can feel this in your bones. Do you feel comfortable around the people you're closest to? Do you have a sort of dull ache in your throat after you've spent an evening or afternoon with a specific person, from wording things in a slightly artificial way or placing your voice somewhere it doesn't naturally sit? When you're socializing with them, do you long to go someplace you can be authentic? Pay close attention. I can't stress enough the importance of having a small, trustworthy inner circle. Feeling that you can be 100 percent yourself around certain people is how you know they're your tribe.

The Nashville Tornado

> Ain't up to me if the sky falls down
> ain't up to me if the lights go out
> every breath, every heartbeat
> you never know where it leads

—"AIN'T UP TO ME"

March 2, 2020, is seared into my memory, because that was the day before everything changed.

The COVID-19 pandemic was beginning to present itself as a potential nationwide crisis in the US. In Nashville, we hadn't even had one case yet; it still felt like something that was happening *elsewhere*, as though it somehow might be contained. I got up, read the news, and tried to put thoughts of this approaching threat from my mind. As I went out into the stunning, crisp, early spring day with my coffee, I saw the most beautiful red bird in my favorite old plum tree. As I looked up, the bird seemed to sing down to me: *It's not up to you—it's out of your control.* I felt a sense of peace as it flew away.

Then I headed to a songwriting session with two writers I hadn't met before, Eric Varnell and Kelli Jones. Because of the pandemic, those of us in the music business were hearing it was likely that tours would soon need to be postponed, and this ended up being our topic of conversation as we settled in and got to know each other.

"Should we write a song called 'Ain't Up to Me'?" I asked. And we did. It was the fastest cowrite I've ever been a part of—the song seemed to write itself as the three of us channeled it.

The rest of the day proceeded as usual. I went home and played with Ernest with his favorite garden hose, because it was his adoptiversary—the date six years earlier that I'd first met him at an adoption event and fallen in love with him. After this, I met producer Bill Reynolds to discuss working together recording songs for my album *The Conduit*, which I was beginning to plan. I then met soul sister Eliza Ann at Bartaco, and returned home.

When it started to rain later that evening, I noticed how the wind was picking up and heard thunder building in the distance. Nothing unusual for Nashville, but as a precaution, I checked the forecast as I got ready for bed. There was a tornado watch, and it was early in the year to have one, but again, nothing unusual for the South. (A "watch" means a tornado *could* form. A "warning" means that a tornado funnel *has* formed and could touch down at any time.)

I couldn't put my finger on it, but something seemed different about this storm. (I'd later hear this same thing from one person after another; a testament to human intuition.) By the time I got into bed after midnight, I felt unusually wary. Ernest was burrowed under the covers against my legs as the storm drew closer. The wind-driven rain was almost as loud as the thunder, and the lightning was so bright it would have kept me awake, so I decided to place an Instacart order for my mom on my phone.

I'm so grateful I had a feeling I shouldn't go to sleep and that my phone was on; I usually set it to airplane mode at bedtime, which would have disabled my storm apps. I was still selecting grocery items when the 4Warn app siren blasted from my phone: "Warning: a tornado has been spotted in your area. Take shelter now."

I summoned Ernest and went down to the basement. We hurried into the place that seemed safest: a dark, windowless room that I'd made into a guest bedroom. The power went out, and suddenly everything got *eerily* silent. I knew then that something bad was about to happen. Ernest and I huddled together, me on my knees with Ernest held tight against me.

Thirty seconds after the power went out, the noise was deafening. It did sound like the rushing rumble of a train I'd always heard accompanies a tornado, but the sound of breaking glass and beams and *everything* from above drowned out the train sound.

There was no question: a tornado had just hit my house.

When the enormous, terrifying noise had faded, and all I could hear was the rain again, I moved to the door and found that I had one bar of service. It was enough to text and make calls, but I definitely couldn't use it to find out what was going on with the storm. Based on what my glimpse of the local weather had been right before losing power, I knew a second tornado could be coming. I was afraid to move.

I called my East Nashville girls and heard they were safe. I also called and texted the neighbors to check on them. When one came over to unlock my door and bring me a pair of shoes before I ventured into the mess (I'd run down in my bare feet), I was astonished to see I still had a roof—a heavily damaged, leaking one, but a roof nonetheless. I was certain it had been entirely ripped off. The windows and the giant trees were almost entirely gone. The fences, gates, carport, garage, siding, shingles, and outdoor structures were tossed into crumpled heaps, as though a giant had trampled through them. The power lines up and down the street were lying in crisscrosses, along with every tree, and debris of all types blanketed properties and pavement alike. Fifteen-foot-high tree-root balls were lying on their sides, extricated from the earth. Houses on my block were completely totaled.

Four houses down, a family with young kids had just gotten everyone up and into the basement at the moment the tornado struck, and their six-year-old's bed ended up in the living room by the piano. Learning from my neighbors as they emerged that everyone was safe was even more impossible to fathom—and nothing short of a miracle.

My insane, incredible friends Fran and Vanessa decided to drive over and get me out of the house for the night. I tried to explain there was no way to get through the debris, but they came anyway without telling me they were doing so. Two blocks away, they couldn't drive any farther, so Vanessa walked to find me. I grabbed Ernest and my computer and whatever I thought I might need. Carrying Ernest, using the light from Vanessa's phone, we made our way over the downed electrical lines (not a good idea!) and to Fran's waiting car. The craziest thing was that only a few blocks away, it looked as though nothing had happened.

Thankfully, Vanessa had power, and we could see on the news how bad it had been. The tornado was later identified as an F3, with 165-mile-per-hour winds. There were multiple tornados in surrounding counties that night, too, and twenty-five people were killed.

As the sun rose, Vanessa settled me into her guest room. The trauma began to hit, so I didn't think I'd be able to sleep. Friends from across the country began waking up to the news of the devastation. My phone blew up with concerned messages, and I didn't want to ignore them. Eventually, I had to turn the phone off, and I slept for a couple of hours. It was a beautiful day and surreal to see the shocking damage juxtaposed against it, in broad daylight.

What impressed me most that day, and in the days that followed, was the extraordinary spirit of Nashville, and specifically East Nashville. This is one of the main reasons I moved to this city in the first place: the indescribable feeling that is more than the love and connection I have for any one person or any few dear friends, but the sense of being *home*. Home in a city that looks after its own.

A few hours later, I returned to my house to find that the massive tree that had fallen across my driveway had been chainsawed down by two of my amazing neighbors (many more of whom I soon got to know). The center of the street was already largely cleared, almost entirely by volunteers. We wouldn't have power for another two weeks, but some of my neighbors had generators; volunteers set up grills and makeshift food and water stations. Over the next six days, strangers by the thousands came out to help.

I was in a bit of a daze, salvaging things in the garage that were destroyed and weeding through the things that weren't. At the same time, I was dealing with insurance to get repairs scheduled and started as soon as possible, and packing what I needed to stay elsewhere. The amount of debris was staggering and overwhelming, yet through it all, all I could think was, *Thank you, thank you, thank you.* It all could have been so much worse.

Those days were completely surreal. Three days after the tornado, I was in my office, gathering my passport and flash drives and other valuables, when the phone rang. It was my literary agent, Todd Shuster, calling from NYC in that excited voice agents only use when they have *very* good news. As I looked outside through a broken window, he told me we had an offer for *Small Changes*—nearly four years after he'd first asked to meet with me to see if I had any ideas for books. The publisher who'd made the winning offer was based in my beloved Nashville, I had met them in person the previous week, and of the ones I'd met with, they had seemed by far the most effortlessly and deeply aligned with my book's intended message. Standing there, about to vacate my home indefinitely, I had to laugh. Tears of gratitude flooded my eyes as I thought, again, of the timing of all of it. How protected I felt, and how full of purpose. My greatest intention with this idea was that it would reach people and help make a difference in their lives. To receive this news at that particular moment, I somehow felt like it was even more affirmation.

I needed a rental that, ideally, would have privacy, a yard for Ernest, and good energy so that I could do a lot of writing. As fate would have it, the perfect accommodation became available, at exactly the right time. The owner of the house, Rita, didn't normally rent her place long-term, but she had a friend she could stay with, and she wanted to help someone who was displaced by the tornado. She loved dogs and had a haven of peace and beautiful energy that Ernest and I felt instantly at home in.

It also bears mentioning that, in the aftermath of rebuilding, there has been an extraordinary energy of rebirth in my neighborhood, with its dear humans who live here. We survived a force of nature that could have caused irreplaceable loss of life. (And we all got the FEMA survivor flyers in our doors to prove it!) The collective gratitude, as well as the determination and community, has only amplified our light.

Strength in the Unexpected

Immediately after the tornado, the first known cases of COVID-19 began to spread in Nashville. Back then, it would have been unfathomable to think of the worldwide disaster that was on its way. Every day brought more conflicting information, fear, and uncertainty, and a sense of isolation that was rooted in more than just not being able to go out and see (or hug) people.

For me, it was a season of true self-reliance. No one but me could change the kind of day I had. No news I read would comfort me or provide any answers—only the opposite, it seemed. The first week or so I was at my rental house, I slept *a lot*. I realized I was still recovering from the shock of the tornado when the reality of COVID-19 set in.

It also wasn't lost on me how different the tornado aftermath would have been if the storm had taken place a few weeks later, when the pandemic shut down everything. The streams of volunteers and the thousands working side by side to help with the cleanup likely wouldn't have been possible.

Through these days, I learned of the strength that lives within two concepts. One: if I believe I'm here for a purpose (I believe all of us are), then I had better fulfill that purpose. I had better wake up every day and care for myself, so I could make the world even a little better, even from isolation. You can best be of service to others when you're first being mindful that your own basic needs are being met. And I needed to take the principles I'd been trying to live by for years and apply them like my life depended on it.

So I made sure to work out every single day—even briefly, even if it would have been easy to sink into despair at the loss and devastation. I took great joy in preparing my meals, because not only were most restaurants closed even for takeout, but because we didn't yet know if it was safe to order food from them.

I fell into a routine. I'd wake up in the morning, drink my celery juice, take my immune-boosting vitamins, and take my good, sweet boy for a walk around the Cherokee Park neighborhood, which we'd been unfamiliar with but fell in love with. I did my best to smile at strangers and acknowledge the unprecedentedly strange times with a warm glance, even as we played sidewalk Frogger to avoid coming within ten feet of anyone. I journaled every night and wrote my dreams most mornings.

The first month or so, I was easy on myself. I sat on the couch and enjoyed my food and a vegan ice cream pint every single night for the first two weeks. I watched TV and documentaries and movies that inspired me and made me laugh and took my mind off everything going on that I couldn't control.

Then, as I felt like the daily mission was no longer simply getting through that day without panicking, and I was coming back to being myself again even though the world outside wasn't, I marveled at the miracle of timing, that I was blessed to have a book to write at this moment. And I took such deep fulfillment in that.

The other thing I learned at this time is that we need each other, and we can continue to connect with each other as deeply, perhaps *even deeper*, through separation.

When my tour that had been scheduled for March–April 2020 was cancelled, as was my time in the studio recording, along with my songwriting sessions, I realized that what I'd miss the most was connecting with others through song. As I started to see artists I admired performing from online platforms, I remembered the shows I'd played years before on StageIt, when I was beginning my career as a singer-songwriter. So I planned a virtual concert from the living room of the rental house.

I'll never forget the feeling after the first show: utter elation, moved to tears at the pure connection. The knowing, despite being one human body in a house alone, that through a computer screen, I had connected to hundreds more, and I could see what they were saying on the message board, and they could see each other too! I felt as high as I've ever felt after the best live shows I've ever done, and even more so in light of the pain and confusion and loneliness we were all feeling. *Together.*

I played fourteen shows that spring, and the greatest blessing of it all was the true friendships that were born through it. About 150 of the beautiful souls who've been most deeply connecting with my music and social media for years now have formed a special club they dubbed my FANily. I can cry just thinking about it. What greater purpose could I possibly ask for? I long to heal hurt and division and bring people together—it's why I make music: to connect in a way that is even deeper than any I've found through speaking. It's the same reason I create characters—hopefully, to bring life to someone you might think you have nothing in common with, but show you she's perhaps more like you than you imagined. To inspire empathy.

During the most challenging times, perhaps it is *our* challenge to rise up and know we can be a beacon of light to everyone around us. But we must care for ourselves *first* in order to do this. I imagine a world where hate is answered by love; where fear is answered by hope; where the flames of violence are answered with peace; where disagreement is answered by discussion, compassion, and openness. No matter what your opinions are, or how vehemently you think you are unlike someone else.

Maybe I'm naïve about this, but I don't want to think so. I do know that it's almost my religion. I believe we're all much more alike than different. And I know that during a time of unprecedented isolation, my FANily and I found connection.

We are in a time of great uncertainty. Whether from a pandemic or political instability or economic woes, all that we can do, all that's in our power, is to celebrate what we've survived and make every day the best we can. If that is simply reminding ourselves, on that day, that we have a purpose— loving ourselves, taking good care of ourselves and not falling apart—that's an accomplishment. If we've survived this much, we can survive another day.

And then there is no telling what we can do.

Finding Your Passions/Hobbies

Our passions are in us for a reason—to point us toward our purpose. Whether or not your passion becomes your vocation, part of why we're here is to make sure we find time to do what we love. No matter how demanding your job or your family commitments, and even if you think you can't possibly figure it out, if only for a few minutes a day, you deserve to do something nourishing and pleasurable for yourself. This will hopefully become one of the most potent small changes you can create in your world.

Pinpointing Your Passions

How do you find the hobbies and activities that make you happy and bring purpose to your life?

The first thing is to *think about what you loved as a child.* Was it art or music, a certain sport, fishing, hiking, designing clothes, or photography? As adults, we remain similar to who we were and what we liked when we were children. I believe that wholeheartedly! I loved playing the piano and acting and creating stories on my typewriter and inventing imaginary worlds with my brother—traits that have served me well in all of the things I do for a living today. I love traveling—meeting new people, seeing new parts of the world or even a new part of a city I already know well. I love hearing people's stories and digging into what makes them tick. And I often have to stop myself from digging too deep so as not to be intrusive or to offer unsolicited advice! That's been me ever since I can remember.

Passions Start Young!

When I first wrote the song "Younger," I was inspired by the idea that who we are when we're very small—our little selves from the ages of four to seven—is the essence of who we are. Then we spend years figuring out who we want to appear as, and devising filters to keep ourselves from showing what we're really feeling and thinking. But if we're lucky, I believe we can get back to the truest version of us we can be.

"Younger" is a love song based on this concept: What if I could connect that little kid version of me to that little kid version of you, and shake off all of the grown-up artifice we've learned to wear that keeps us from connecting the rest of the way?

Let's run where it says there is no running
let's break our hearts open wide
turn down the static and the buzzing
let's leave this cage and lose our chains

The second thing to do is ask yourself: *What most resonates with my need for self-expression and fulfillment right now?* Only you can answer that, of course, but I'm always amazed at how many people I've met who are stumped when I ask them about their hobbies or what they like to do in their spare time. Many of them don't believe they *have* spare time, but they spend a whole lot of it watching TV they don't even enjoy, or glued to social media. I've experienced that myself!

What if, instead of flipping through TV channels for several hours, you read a book about something you've been meaning to learn more about? Or spend a little time learning a new language? For example, there's a language app called Duolingo that I've always deeply enjoyed when I open it. I just forget it's there sometimes! It works for me because it's fun and doesn't feel like lessons, and it's organized into game-like activities. Or learn an instrument—not because it's something you plan to do professionally, but because it's fun to be able to pick out the notes to one of your favorite songs. I love to noodle on the guitar when I have spare time. This makes it feel more like a pastime and less like, *Oh, I ought to learn this because then I could write some songs on the guitar and make this part of my profession.*

A huge part of my own small-changes manifesto is my passion for three things:

creating music, growing food, and loving/being loved by my rescue animals. Songwriting is about creating something tangible and sing-along-able—from my point of view about something I think I can best express in music form—and then sharing it with the world, in the hope that other people will find that it perfectly describes how they feel but didn't have the words for. Sharing your life with animals is a life-changing experience that enriches you beyond any measure—you nurture them, and they nurture you back in countless, magical ways. And being able to nourish yourself with produce you grew from tiny seeds, in your own soil, in your own back yard? I get giddy just thinking about it. That reminds me: I have this year's first harvested sweet potato sitting on the counter, cooling from the oven. I'd best go cut it open and see if it's delicious!

The Joys of My Music

As you know now, playing the piano has been an integral part of my life since I first placed my hands on the keys, and in chapter 1, I described how I became a prolific songwriter. I'm certain that my first ache to not leave Nashville was also steeped in the music—in knowing that spending time here was key to me discovering the voice I was meant to develop in telling stories through song. Even writing on my own, back in LA where I still lived, felt freer when I began going back and forth to Nashville.

Inspiration finds me wherever I turn—especially the sense that everyone around me is doing the same thing, and in this vibrant musical community, many have been, for generations.

When I search for examples of what making music has meant to me over the years, many memories flood my heart. One forever memory is the night I made my debut at the Grand Ole Opry. At that time, in 2016, I was still prone to butterflies at live shows, yet it astonished me how calm and present I felt once I walked onto that hallowed stage. I knew it was because of all the spirits, alive and passed, who had filled the space with their gift and their grace. There were 4,400 people there that night, by far the largest crowd I'd ever played to, and I looked out at them and felt pure peace and exhilaration. I knew that whatever happened going forward with my music, that night was proof I belonged in that world.

Singing and playing with the Opry Band backing me up, and some of my dearest friends—along with my lifelong biggest fans, my mom and dad—in the audience, I felt that I'd never again be nervous singing in front of a crowd. Which wasn't true. I remember being shocked at a tiny show in LA the next year, when I felt so nervous I could barely catch my breath for the first few songs! But what is true is that I can go back to that place in my mind whenever I want to. And in moments when I do feel those butterflies, whether in a music capacity or otherwise, I remember the feeling of being supported during my Opry performance, and I know I'm in my purpose. And I know I won't be given any task I can't handle. Also, the Opry never would have happened if I hadn't spent all those hours upon countless tens of thousands of hours sitting alone at my piano, figuring out how to tell stories there because something compelled me to do it.

What in your own life does this remind you of? What do you imagine yourself doing and excelling at, just for the fun of it, but haven't found the time for yet? Whatever comes to mind first, I bet you're on to it.

The Joys of My Garden

I've always wanted to have a farm. As a five-year-old, when asked what I wanted to be when I grew up, one of my intended vocations was "farmstress." I think part of that early desire to live off my land came from having adored the Little House books by Laura Ingalls Wilder as a child. The idea of going out to my backyard, picking what I needed for my meal, and preparing it has always filled me with a feeling that can only be described as glee. I tried to the best of my ability to make this dream a reality at my home in LA, but the land was uncooperative. Plus, I had a bumper crop of snails that were undeterred by beer traps or handpicking at dusk. There were hundreds of them every night, in the spring and summer.

I am lucky to have enough space in my Nashville backyard for a wonderful garden, and to have a space in which fruits and veggies love to grow. When I first saw this house, one of the biggest selling points for me was the (then) rickety raised-bed planter out in the back, which was overflowing with overgrown, but blissfully happy, veggies. Peppers, tomatoes, greens—they weren't even being looked after, yet they flourished. That was a sign. The large vegetable garden in another area of the yard hadn't been tilled or propagated in years, but I set to work on that the first spring I was there, and I've been learning by leaps and bounds ever since. But it's not all me, by any means: this space wants to grow veggies. I only give them what they need, and they jump for joy. It's not lost on me that it's become a miniature version of what I envisioned when I first read *Little House on the Prairie*.

I get so much joy out of harvesting my own vegetables and preparing a meal for friends based on ingredients I grew myself. It's deeply pleasurable to know you were responsible for turning a few tiny seeds and plants into something edible and nutritious. It's also quite meditative to check on the fruits of your labors. Watching your garden grow and nurturing it and then seeing it fulfill its purpose—to propagate, or be eaten, or both—is amazingly soul-satisfying. Ernest would be the first to agree. He loves his fruits and veggies, and he does seem to especially savor a treat when I've just picked it off one of our plants. (His favorite is watermelon, although he'll eat nearly anything. He also enjoys being given a giant stalk of kale or collard greens and fastidiously tearing it into confetti strips!)

Even if you live in a city apartment or home without access to space for an outdoor garden, you can still nurture your green thumb with an indoor garden. There's nothing more enticing in a kitchen than pots of herbs in the window, and they're ridiculously easy to grow. With a little extra love, many vegetables can be grown in pots.

On my rare days completely off (translation: the rare days when I decide to take the entire day off), I'm often in the garden from 7:00 a.m. till the sun goes down, harvesting and weeding and fertilizing and planting and spraying for bugs (organic only) and bringing the crops in, then washing, chopping, and flash-freezing them if I've got a surplus, cooking with them, and then happily eating my homegrown creations. Wearing a wide sombrero and sunscreen, working all day in the great outdoors, and then going to bed exhausted but satisfied, is one of my favorite ways to enjoy a day. And I'm not ashamed to admit that when I travel, whether for fun or for work, I truly miss my garden.

In addition, one of the best benefits to heavy-duty gardening is how labor intensive it is, especially with the size of the weeds we can get here in Nashville! I swear those things pop up seemingly overnight. Not only is gardening fun and interesting, but if you spend the entire day doing it, it's a real workout, particularly for your glutes, core, and upper body. I love to find a great audiobook or podcast series and listen while I garden. Even on days when I have a lot of work to do, I try to take a break for time in the garden, even if it's only fifteen minutes of picking a few things or making a batch of pesto from fresh-picked basil and saving it for later.

So what all do I grow? Collard greens, kale, arugula, zucchinis, sweet potatoes, corn, cucumbers, broccoli, eggplants, okra, peas, squashes, watermelons, peppers, heirloom and cherry tomatoes, blueberries, and strawberries. I also plant pretty much every herb that grows well in this region, along with onions and garlic. Did you know you can plant the root end of a garlic clove in the ground and then forget about it, and by the end of the year, a whole bulb will be ready to dig up? Onions and garlic also help repel some bugs—as do marigolds, if you plant enough of them. I haven't mastered the art of keeping all pests off by using nothing but plants, but if you can't already tell, I could spend all day, every day learning about this!

Sweet potatoes have, likewise, turned into a pseudo-obsession, as you'll see in the recipe for Sweet Potato Soup on page 217 in chapter 9. I also have peach, cherry, plum, pear, and apple trees that survived the tornado, which heartbreakingly uprooted nearly all of the enormous, decades-old trees in the neighborhood. And I found a couple of varieties of fig tree that can survive our Zone 7 winters with extra protection in the form of burlap. They've already been producing delicious figs in their first few months being in the ground, and I can't wait to watch them grow.

The first few springs I lived here, I made jars and jars of plum preserves since they all ripen nearly at once, and it's gratifying to wake up on a chilly morning months later and be able to spread that sweet, homegrown, spring-time flavor on a piece of toast. That tree split in the tornado, but I cried tears of relief when I saw that the remaining half was salvageable, after the broken parts were pruned off and the open wounds were sealed. It was in shock, but it did produce a nice mini crop of delicious plums for me a few months after the tornado.

The Joys of My Furry Friends

A small change for you can make a huge difference for an animal in need! Not only are you saving another life and making the world a better place, but you're giving yourself a gift that can never be measured.

This is why I always encourage animal lovers to turn to their local shelter or rescue facility when they're considering a new pet. You can find puppies, purebreds, or mixed breeds; there are also countless breed-specific rescue groups, and many of them have volunteers who will drive an animal across the country if need be to match them with the right family. Not much is more wonderful than seeing a scared animal taken out of a shelter and blossom with love in a new home.

If you're worried about an animal acting out due to previous abuse or neglect, which is an especially valid concern for families with young children, you can adopt from an organization like Take Me Home. They rescue dogs from kill shelters in the LA area and then place them with foster guardians in homes, so they can be carefully observed as their personalities emerge. This minimizes any surprises about potential behavioral issues. Organizations like these can be found in almost any state or municipality.

I've had four rescues so far: three dogs and a feral cat. Through them, as well as all of my friends' animal companions I've grown close to over the years, I've learned that all animals are unique. They pick up your energy, without question. But beyond that, they all have a spirit and a soul and an individual personality, and the more time you spend around them, the deeper you see them and the more you love them. I can't begin to measure the ways that my animals have improved my life, with their boundless understanding and goofy wonderfulness.

Sometimes, when I come home to a hotel room after work, I'd collapse and go right to bed, if not for needing to take Ernest for a walk. (Which is a great way to wind down and decompress after a long day.) Other times when I'm home, or in a rental house with a backyard, I could easily just let him out to do his "business," but he always knows when *I* need to go out to clear my head. I swear he does! Just last night, in the midst of writing this book, I was feeling groggy, processing the changing of the seasons and feeling chilled and sniffly. Not a good headspace to be in during the age of COVID-19. When I went to open the back door for him, Ernest pawed at me and didn't want to just be let out—he wanted me to join him for a dusk walk. And you guessed it: I felt 100 percent better after we did that together! His head is resting on my leg as I write this. (To be clear, he's also hoping to lick my plate when I'm done eating my veggie sausage, broccoli, and spinach with pesto.)

Animals are also remarkable for their ability to exist primarily in the here and now—reminding us to do the same—but I don't agree with the notion that they can't understand the concept of time. I've always spoken to mine in complete sentences, explaining what we're about to do or who's coming over; I've seen them fill with anticipation, waiting by the door, completely unsurprised when the event I described happens. When I lived in LA, a ten-minute drive from a beautiful hike where I could take my dogs off leash, I'd tell them, "Tomorrow morning, we're gonna go to Mountaingate!" and they'd wake me with the sun, knowing what was about to happen in a specific, expectant way. Conversely, it's incredible to watch the way they don't think about anything other than what they're experiencing in the moment—and how quickly they tend to "shake it off" when something happens to them that isn't fun. As people, we tend to primarily live within a constant narrative that's racing through our minds, and it's easy to forgot how lucky we are to be here.

My Favorite Dog Training Tip

I've shared this with all of my friends when they've adopted a dog, as it works like a charm. Simply tie a dangling bird toy with bells to each door that you want your puppy to use when going out to do their business. Whenever you take the little one outside, be sure the bell rings as you open the door. Within a few days, you'll have your puppy ringing the bell to go out!

How I Met My Ernest

After my beloved Jessie (feral tabby cat) and Jake (red rescue dog) passed away at ripe old ages within five days of each other, my remaining dog, Maggie, was in shock. She'd been the baby of the family, and now she was the only animal. I was heartbroken to hear from a neighbor that she'd howled for hours the first day I went back to work on *Justified*. Even when I brought her to the set with me, I could tell her heart wasn't in it. It was time to find her the perfect new companion.

My friend Jessika had adopted two amazing rescues from Take Me Home. Maggie and I went to one of their adoption events with Jess, and the founder, Haze, pointed out a ten-month-old puppy, standing off to the side with his foster mom. He'd been adopted at seven months, then returned two months later to the West LA kill shelter with no reason given (having lost two of his only fourteen pounds at the time!). He was still undergoing worm treatments, so he couldn't be with the other dogs yet. Once in a while he would try, then, realizing he was held back by his leash, he patiently sat back down in his spot next to the foster mom. His zen attitude was striking, especially in a dog so young. I instantly couldn't get him out of my head.

The next weekend, I planned to visit him again with Maggie, to see if they were a good match, and I brought my then-boyfriend Ben's kids with me to have a say. I mentioned that we were also on a name-seeking mission. He'd already been through a few names in his journey so far, and he needed a brand-new name for his brand-new life.

A few blocks away from the adoption event, we all remarked on a bearded man who looked just like Ernest Hemingway, riding a bicycle down Venice Beach. Then we pulled up, got out, and met my sweet boy. Within fifteen seconds of seeing him for the first time, Ben's daughter Gracie said, "I think his name might be Ernest." I instantly knew his name could never be anything else!

When Maggie and Ernest met that day, they were curious and relaxed with each other, as if they'd always been acquainted. On his first day home, Ernest gathered all of Maggie's toys and brought them one by one onto the couch, and then settled himself up there, too, falling asleep surrounded by them. Maggie didn't mind at all. They immediately became best friends, and Ernest's love and youthful energy cured her of her grief and depression.

It was incredible to watch Maggie, the forever puppy, turn into a mama bear for Ernest in her later years. The other thing that was a marvel right away was that Ernest went to each of Jake's specific favorite spots and adopted them as his own, as though Jake's energy was leading him there. He even adopted Jake's favorite patch of driveway for sunning himself out front, which, three months after Jake's passing, couldn't realistically have smelled like him any longer.

A year and a half later, only a few days after Maggie left us, I had to fly out of town for my next shoot, filming the Hallmark movie *I'm Not Ready for Christmas* (named after my song!), and Ernest and I healed the loss as we flew off on our new adventure together. Ernest's first plane ride was a dream, as if he'd been flying all his life. His eyes got big when he looked out the window at the clouds, and he never made a peep. It's been such a gift to see him grow into his role as my only dog.

Ernest is now my near-constant companion on film and TV sets, in recording studios, and on airplanes. His empathic and peaceful energy brings grateful tears to my eyes on a daily basis. And his presence also brings lots of short, black hairs the wardrobe department is constantly lint-rolling off of my clothes. So worth it, and they agree; he makes friends on every single set.

> Animals are there for you, and with you, in your most private of moments. They know you so well, yet without ever having the gift of speaking in words. Perhaps that's why they know you so well—they don't have the gift of miscommunication that we humans seem to excel at.

You might think you're not ready for a pet, but once that furry friend arrives, you won't be able to imagine life without them. I know I will adopt again, since I loved the camaraderie of having a whole animal family running around the house and watching their relationships with each other, as well as with me. But for the time being, I'm loving the flexibility and partnership of having just Ernest. Practically speaking, it's much easier to bring one animal on work trips than more than one, or to leave him at a friend's home for a few days and return the favor when they need a sitter for their dog. When I had a menagerie, anything except a multi-monthlong job meant hiring a house sitter to live at my house with the three of them.

Whether you choose to bring a rescued best friend into your life or not, I hope that whatever passions engage your spirit will bring you as much joy as my animals have brought me. Rescue animals enrich lives in ways that I've tried to share on these pages—and learning to amplify my own light and love through loving these deserving animals has been one of the greatest small changes in my life.

CHAPTER 6

Finding Yourself in the Silence

You have the choice to

Reveal the quiet that you're hiding in your voice

—"YOUNGER"

Having a healthy inner life isn't just about finding your passions and your balance. For me, it's also about finding myself in the silence—doing the deep introspective work that gives me confidence in who I am and ensures that I stay close to my most authentic self.

This chapter will delve into the life-affirming power of meditation and journaling. I've incorporated these practices into my life and use them to stay level-headed, calm, and grateful for every moment—and you can too. It's my wish for you to walk away from this chapter with a new perspective on just how helpful these practices can be and how easily you can implement them into your everyday life, no matter how busy you are. They're a perfect example of how a small change—a commitment to trying something new for a few minutes each day—can lead to big, positive results and make you a happier, more balanced person.

The Power of Meditation

I've found that many people are intimidated by meditation, thinking they'll do it wrong or that they have to become a full-on Buddhist or yogi to embrace the practice. I'm happy to clear up this misconception!

I first learned about meditation in the book *Wherever You Go, There You Are* by Jon Kabat-Zinn. My biggest takeaway from it remains the section on simple meditation: focusing on your breath going in for a certain count, your breath going out for a certain count, pausing for a few seconds, and then repeating the sequence. When thoughts come up, you try to calm yourself through your breath. That's basic meditation, and this kind of breathing helps you slow things down, so you can cope better.

About ten years ago, I was gifted a training in Transcendental Meditation, or TM. In this practice, you're given a mantra—not meant to be shared or said aloud—which is based on what you're trying to accomplish with your meditation. There's something incredibly peaceful about that mantra, and the knowledge that whenever you silently repeat it, the only thing on your mind will be going to that peaceful place. When thoughts come up, you don't force them away, but rather observe them, like little thought bubbles, as you refocus on your mantra. By doing this, and doing it every day, you can become more aware of what thoughts you want to include in your life. This not only helps great ideas come to you with more frequency, but you can start to see erratic behavior, like when you have an impulse to do something you know you shouldn't, or when your brain starts spinning out over someone else's actions.

TM brings whatever is at your core to the forefront and helps shine a light on it. Then, if what you see is something you wish to transform, TM can help to do that in a big way. It won't change who you are intrinsically though. It simply helps bring you back to who you are at the core.

A few years back, I was experiencing disillusionment with TM, upon learning that someone I knew was still engaging in the same addictive patterns he'd sworn TM had healed him of. A teacher who helped reconnect me with my practice used this analogy: if you're a bank robber, TM will make you the *best* bank robber you can be. I loved that explanation. Once meditation ends, it's up to you what you choose to do with the illumination you receive from it. It does have the power to *help you* break a cycle that has held you prisoner your whole life. But that decision is yours.

While I love what I get from TM, I don't practice it as regularly as its teachers would instruct, which is twenty minutes twice a day. Many people who are exceptionally busy do find the time, so it's not merely because of that. I find it helpful even if I do that particular discipline of meditation only once in a while, or for a short period. I don't think it's either twice a day or not at all. And although you're not technically *supposed* to use it to fall asleep, some of my most incredible sleeps have occurred in the midst of a late-night meditation. (This is the no-rules gal you're talking to, after all.) Regardless of the form of meditation, some type of daily meditation is essential for me now. I really notice when I don't do it!

I've gotten some of my best ideas—without trying to "think" of them—following or even during a meditation. I've given myself reminders about jobs I want to follow up on and reached out immediately after I came out of meditating, to discover that the timing was uncanny. Many of the ideas and concepts I wanted to put forth for this book became crystallized during a meditation. Songs have been finished (or conceptualized entirely), and I even figured out how to set up my living room in my Nashville home—I realized I could move my pull-out sofa, which was smack-dab in the middle of the living room, into the corner by the dining table. Then I could pull out the bed for houseguests, who'd feel as though they were in a private-ish area and not in the middle of the living room. Now, I didn't *do* exactly that, but the idea led me to the setup I currently have and started me revisualizing the whole flow of the space.

How to Meditate

Many people erroneously think that meditation has to be long and complicated to be beneficial, so they put off doing it because they don't think they have the time. However, you can meditate for a mere three minutes a day, and it *will* make a difference!

Start slow. There's a time and place for doing something small every day. Try it for three or five minutes and see how it feels. An easy way to do this is to meditate for a few minutes every morning, before you get out of bed or turn on your phone. Set your alarm for ten minutes earlier than you need to wake up. Taking those moments to connect to your own thoughts is incredibly helpful. If you can meditate for five minutes, you might find that when the time ends, you're just getting started. You then might want to go for ten minutes, or maybe you'll get to a deeper place if you go for fifteen minutes.

I often like to meditate while doing a twenty-minute free-flow yoga session. Sometimes, quiet meditation isn't always best because your mind starts to wander, and some of us end up being more mentally active when we're sitting still. Combining meditation with yoga gives me the benefits of both, and I always leave each session refreshed and energized. If you're trying this, I'd suggest adding a mantra (see below) or doing your free-flow session using a timed meditation app (like the Oprah/Deepak one, which I also reference below).

FINDING YOUR MEDITATION PLACE

Because my workplaces and schedules are constantly shifting, I've learned how to meditate (and eat!) just about anywhere.

When I'm on a set, I'm typically provided with a driver, and I like to meditate in the car on the way to work. I also love to do this on public transportation, like on the subway or an airplane. Takeoffs and landings are fantastic meditation settings. You can even do it in the pickup line at school, if you have a bit of a wait for the kids. I've meditated in my dressing room and often do it while I'm being tended to in the hair and makeup chair. You can also meditate in a doctor's waiting room, during a break at work, while you're waiting for your dinner to cook, on a blanket on the grass or on a bench outside. There's nothing quite like tuning out the world while you're surrounded by it, and simultaneously connecting deeper to it, through connecting to your inner self.

Make a Mantra Your Own

Mantras can be thought of as affirmations and are often related to specific things we need to work on, whether in relationships with other people or with aspects of our behavior or health. You can create a mantra for yourself and repeat it fifty times while you're breathing in and out. That will only take about five to ten minutes. Usually, you don't say the mantra out loud; you just think it.

Choosing the perfect mantra for the moment is powerful. I usually do this when I'm sitting under a special tree in my garden. But I also have several short sentences and sayings I use on a regular basis for meditation. These are deeply personal mantras for me. Affirming them silently leaves me centered and connected to what I believe my purpose to be. Whatever mantra you feel is right for you at any point in time, probably is. As you use them, you'll feel your own inner knowledge taking shape.

Using Guided Meditations

Guided meditations are helpful and inspiring as well, and there are countless options online. Listening to a soothing voice can quickly lull you into that perfect meditative state and help you to figure out what kinds of meditation work best for you. You can find many free meditation apps on your phone, such as Calm, which has a wide array of timed meditations, both spoken and either sound- or music-based, geared specifically to the goals you're most interested in.

I particularly like the Oprah/Deepak twenty-one-day meditation courses. Once you buy them, they're yours forever. Each meditation lasts twenty minutes, which includes an intro in Oprah's loving, empathic voice; an eight-minute talk on the subject of the day in Deepak's healing, peaceful one; a mantra to use during that day's meditation; and an intention of the day. I find these perfect when set to a brief yoga flow, as well as before falling asleep or anytime really. Two of my favorites of these courses are *Finding Your Flow* and *Energy of Attraction: Manifesting Your Best Life.* I have such better days when I make the time to do them.

Using Meditation When You're Tired

When I was making a movie recently, working on too little sleep for three nights straight, my head started spinning. I was thinking I appeared worse than I actually did and finding myself angsting over certain relationships that my gut told me were no longer healthy for me. I found fault with everyone and everything while trying to contain my negative feelings. It took all of my willpower not to text those people and tell them how I was feeling, because I always want to be transparent and honest. This wasn't transparency though—it was *exhaustion.*

When you're feeling extra moody and anxious and stressed, it's a good idea to ask yourself if you've gotten enough sleep. Go easy on yourself and admit that you haven't allowed yourself to recharge! Realizing that this feeling will pass can help the nasty mood dissipate sooner. Then use this realization to

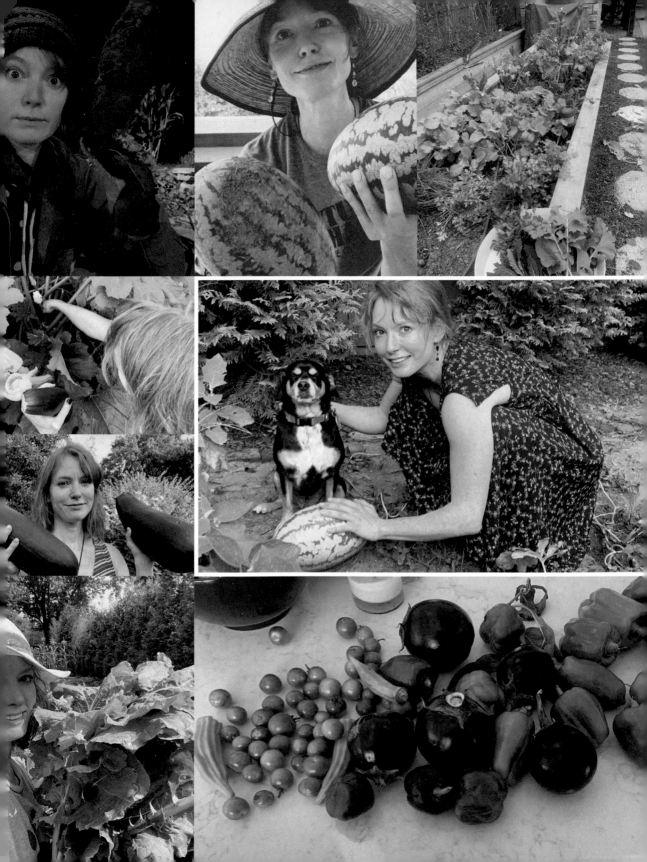

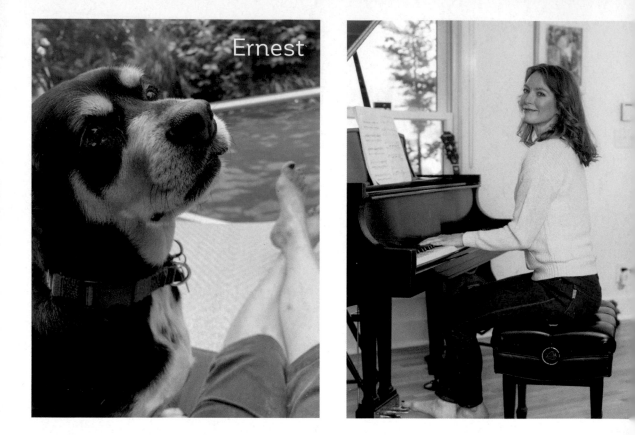
Ernest

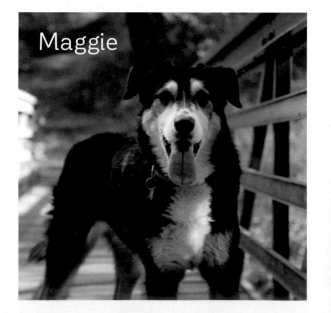
Maggie

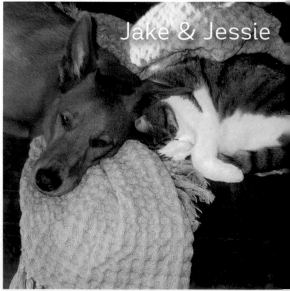
Jake & Jessie

The Joys of My Life: Music, Gardening & Furry Friends

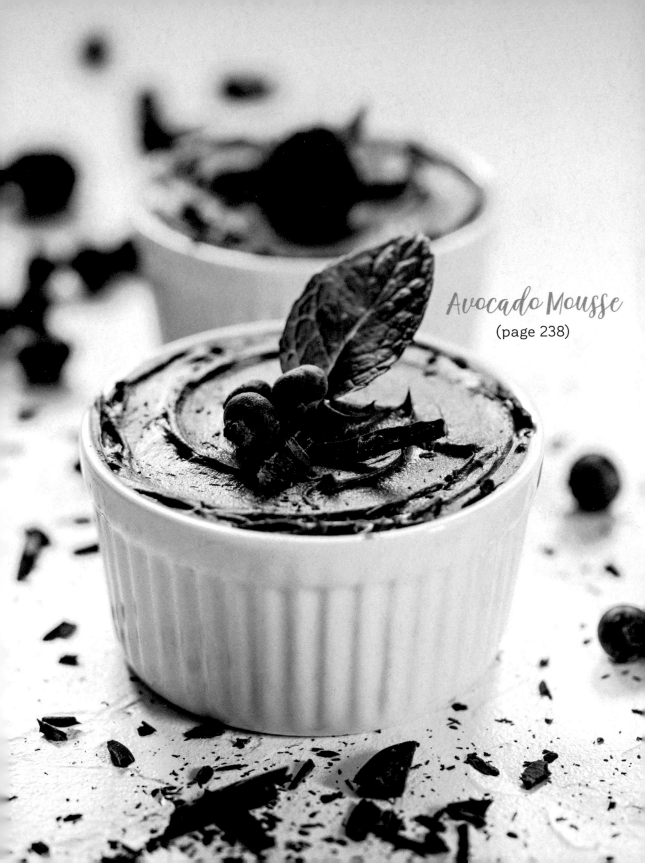

Avocado Mousse
(page 238)

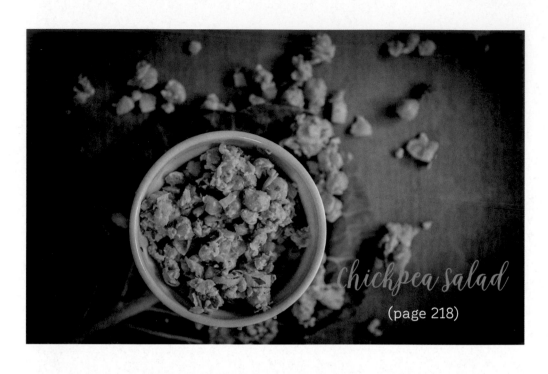

chickpea salad
(page 218)

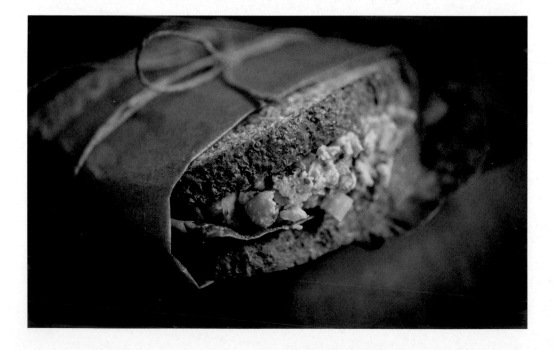

Creamy Mushroom Pasta

(page 222)

Gazpacho

(page 215)

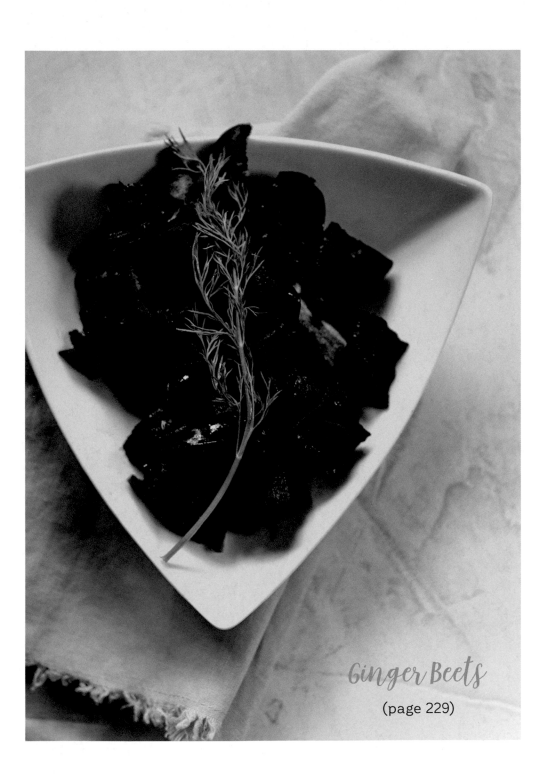

Ginger Beets

(page 229)

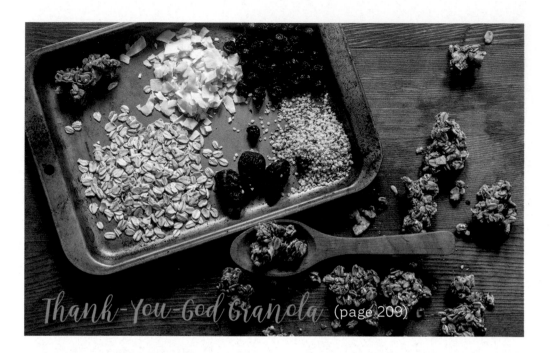

Thank-You-God Granola (page 209)

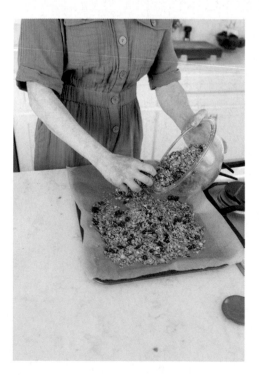

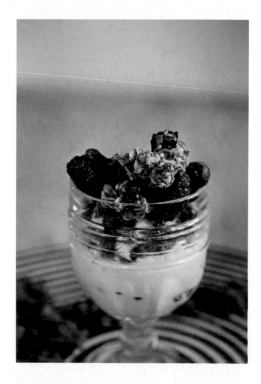

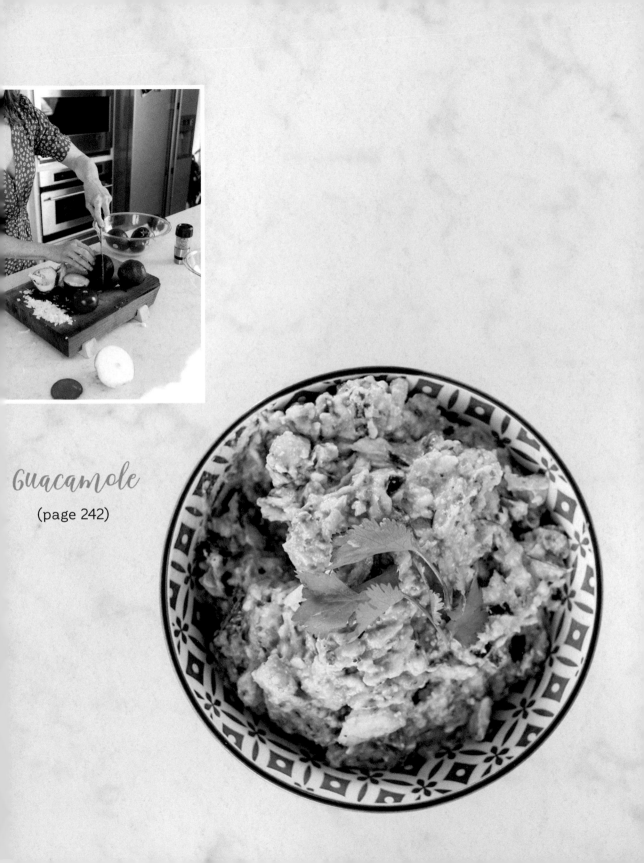

Guacamole

(page 242)

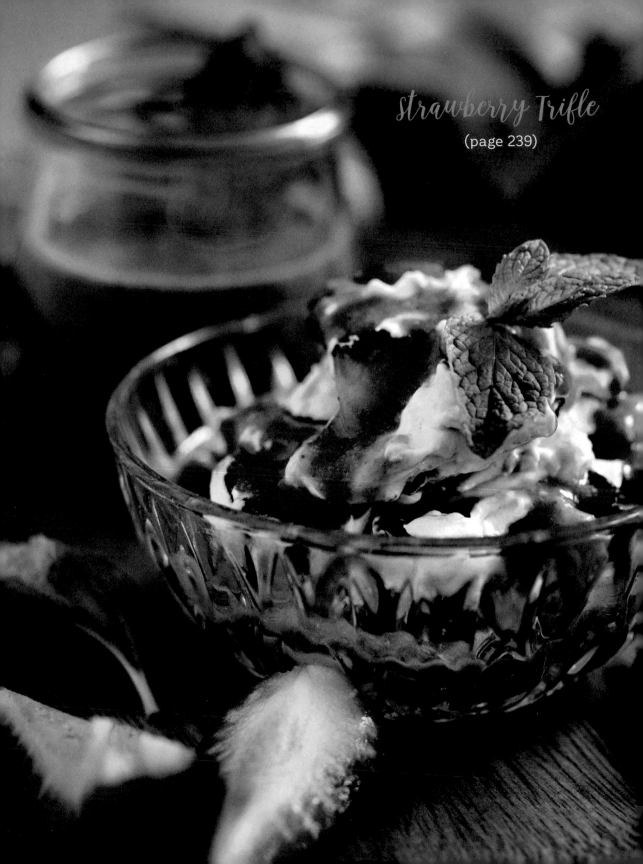

strawberry Trifle

(page 239)

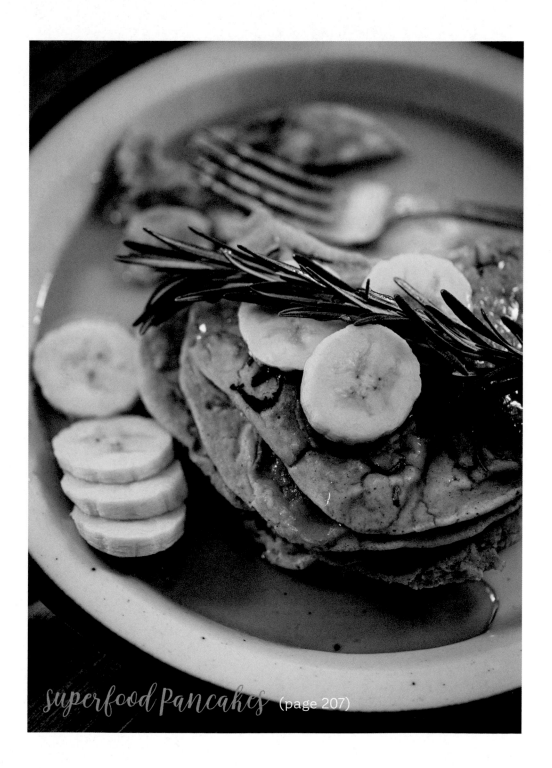

superfood pancakes (page 207)

Zucchini Lasagna
(page 235)

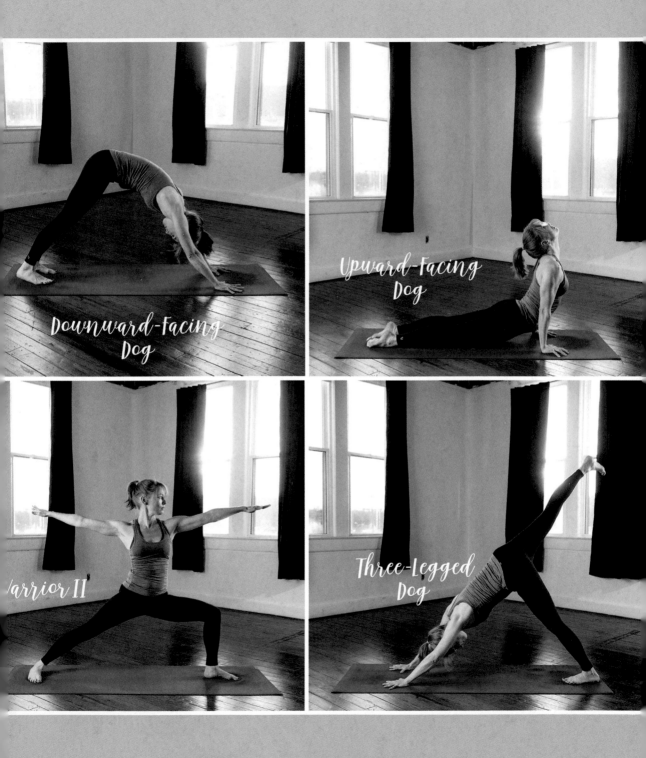

Downward-Facing Dog

Upward-Facing Dog

Warrior II

Three-Legged Dog

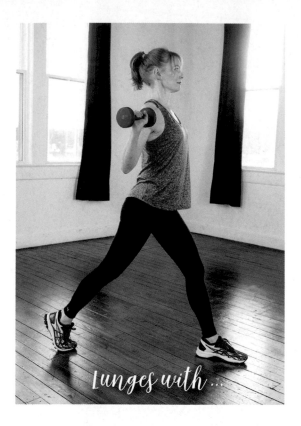

Lunges with ...

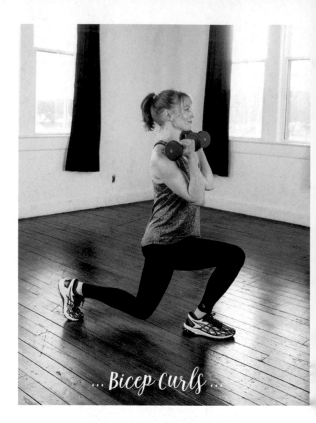

... Bicep Curls ...

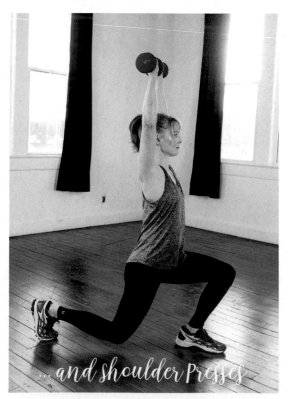

... and Shoulder Presses

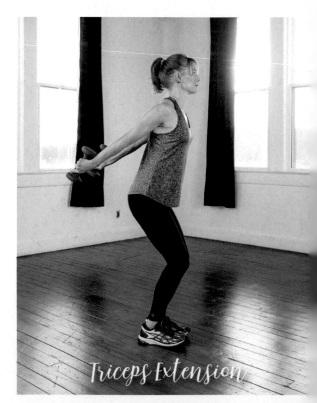

Triceps Extension

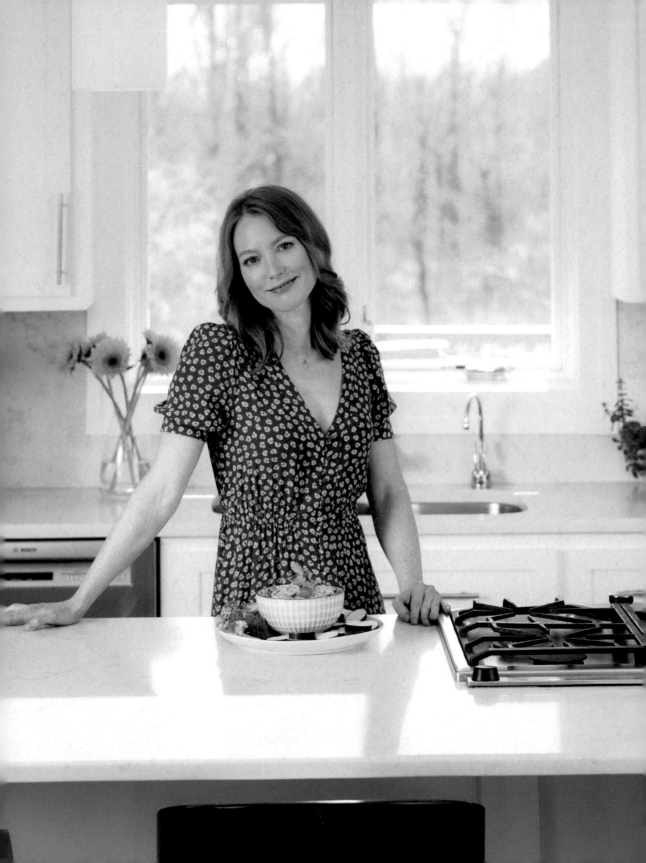

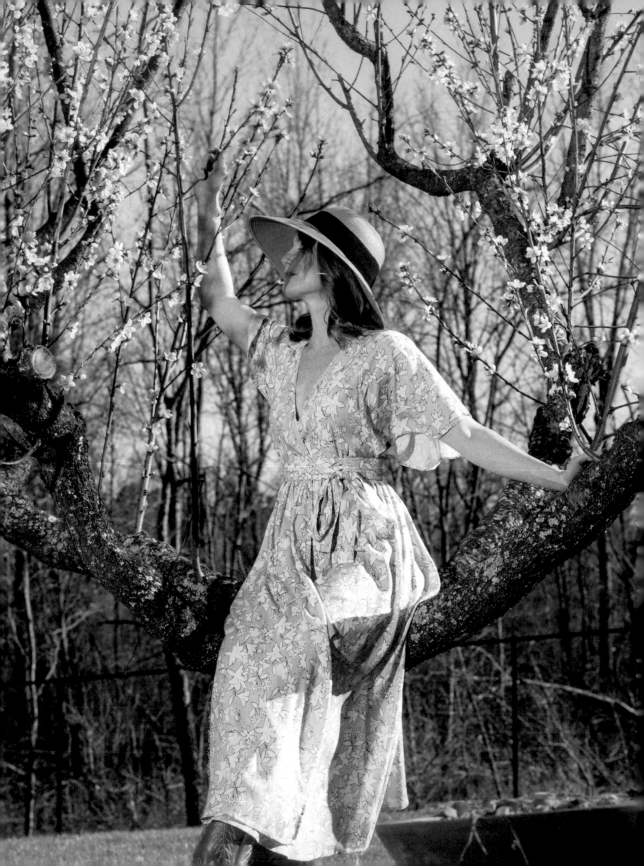

relax and spend a few minutes in meditation, to clear your head and return you to a sense of accomplishment and perspective.

Setting Intentions

There's something about clearing your mind during morning meditation that makes it easier to identify your intentions for the day.

On New Year's Eve, I don't create a list of "will do every day/will never do again" resolutions anymore—I think this sets you up for failure. Instead, I write extensively about what the year taught me and what I'd like the next year to bring. This has been vastly rewarding, and I'm blown away by how much happened that year and filled with awe and inspiration for the year ahead, as midnight draws close.

Daily intentions are equally satisfying. It's like doing a mental or emotional exercise—a self-soothing, self-empowerment practice that's easy when you think of the process as taking baby steps as opposed to running a marathon.

Setting simple, doable intentions helps keep your mind as healthy as your body. This is something I learned to do as an actor, because I need to set the intentions for a fictional character in order to better play the role. For example, I'll create playlists for certain characters—like Zelda, as she was feeling drawn to complicated Piper on *Orange Is the New Black*—to help me get inside what a character is feeling. If I'm working out in the morning while I'm in the midst of that job, I might listen to that playlist and think of how I'll play certain scenes, or transport myself into that mindset. But at the same time, I need to not *lose myself* in the role or alternate universe, and remain grounded in my own intentions and my own life while embodying someone else. I often get ideas during the days off from a job like that, which I write down and try out when I'm at work.

What I absolutely *don't* want is to apply my character's angst to my own life. I do the work in advance and set those intentions, so I know what I can call on from my own history and my character's invented history in those moments, so that then they can surprise me and hopefully create a living, breathing experience, captured forever on film. Isn't this so true of real life as well? Set the intentions, and then just be present.

I had a forever lesson in this notion from the irreplaceable Al Pacino. No one was more surprised than I was to be cast in the lead role opposite him in *88 Minutes* in 2005. I had a great first audition with director Jon Avnet, and he asked if I'd stick around for a table read-through of the script that Al was coming in to do later. That was already more than I could have dreamed of, and I hunkered down in an empty room at Jon's offices to familiarize myself with my many lines and to try to calm my pounding heart.

When I was a teenager going to Blockbuster Video to rent three movies a night for a crash course in this business I hoped to make a mark in, Al became one of my earliest acting influences. It may not be readily apparent from watching *Fun*, but I'm sure I wouldn't have come up with that performance if I hadn't been inspired by Al's fearless one in *Dog Day Afternoon*. He's one of the first actors who took my breath away and made me think, *This is what I moved out to LA to do.* And now I was going to spend two hours reading scene after scene opposite him, for an entire script!

From the moment I shook his hand that afternoon, I stopped being nervous around him. He was that grounded, that much just a *human being*—an actor still striving to do great work, even in a popcorn thriller. I got to know Al well during many private flights he invited me to share, between our location in Vancouver and LA, where his young kids lived. He also impressed upon me the most extraordinary work ethic I'd ever seen, especially in light of his goes-without-saying legendary status. He's the kind of actor who will ask to do a dialogue-free scene crossing the street seven times if he thinks he can improve his performance, not because he's flexing an ego.

Each weekend he took the cast members scheduled to work that week, and Avnet, out to a private dinner at his favorite Italian restaurant in Vancouver.

We would read through our upcoming scenes and improvise—discussing in detail the characters' motivations and making changes as we went along—for a script that would likely never be the most critically acclaimed entry on any of our résumés. Still, as much as I grew to love and feel comfortable around my *friend* Al, I couldn't get away from the truth that I was acting directly opposite the *legend* Al. I wanted to give the role 110 percent.

This was never more apparent than when it came time for us to film the scene where our characters, Jack and Kim, show up at the apartment of one of the murder victims. Kim, a forensic psychiatry graduate student, has never seen an actual crime scene, and when they discover this young woman's remains, Kim loses it. That's what was scripted. And, man oh man, was I determined to deliver!

We rehearsed the scene, and I asked (as I still would today) to be kept from accidentally glimpsing the actor playing the dead woman when she was brought to set after her special effects makeup was applied, wanting to see it for the first time with cameras rolling. Al went to get a coffee and relax, and I sat in a corner on the set, not looking at or talking to anyone, psyching myself up for the big moment. At my request, we weren't going to rehearse again once they got the cameras set up but would film the first take.

We started rolling. We walked in the door, guns drawn, and rounded the corner, and when I/Kim saw the "corpse," I had an out-of-body experience. I started shaking and sweating and crying and hyperventilating so hard I couldn't function. I forgot where I was—I *became* Kim in that moment. I couldn't say a line or continue with the scene as we'd rehearsed it. Heck, I forgot we were filming. Al had to slap me twice on the face to snap me out of it! Not a painful slap—a solid, *wake up!*, cupped-hand slap like you'd give to a victim who had passed out. And it worked! I came back to him and finished the scene, catching my breath enough to remember what I was supposed to say and do.

As they set up for the next take, Al and I went over to our seats to wait.

After a few moments of silence, in which I was thinking I had done something impressive, Al spoke to me in a quiet voice.

"You know, you don't have to do that much. You don't have to get that worked up for a scene like this," he said kindly, not talking down—just honest.

"What do you mean?" I asked, stunned.

"The way they edit it—it's all these little pieces, and sound effects. It's all in the rhythm of it. As long as you get all those pieces right, the scene will work."

He wasn't trying to lecture me. He wanted to spare me a lifetime of doing what I'd just done, thinking that was how to deliver the best performance. I didn't need to go into deep method acting (or whatever my untrained idea of method acting is) for what would ultimately be a brief scene in an action thriller. My mind instantly flashed to all the times I'd done something so similar, in similar scenes.

> Just because you feel like you're working as hard as you possibly can doesn't necessarily make the work better.

Sure enough, that take, proud as I still am of it, is *not* in the movie. It would have been way too much! At that point, the movie is racing toward its finish and the audience should be trying to figure out who's trying to kill Jack, not taking a detour into Kim's psychological state. I learned more that day than years of acting classes could have taught me. Since then, it's been so freeing to know that, whether it's an action scene that flashes by or a deeply emotional moment, I can jump into whatever state of mind I need to, then jump right back out of it again. And it's better and fresher when I do it that way than if I plan and plot and immerse myself to the point where I can't be me in between takes. It gives me the space to play and discover in the moment—and to be more fully present both while I'm working, and when the work ends.

Again, a beautiful life lesson.

Whatever line of work you're in, it's important to take even a few breaths of time in the morning, to focus on the intention you want to set for the day.

Do you have a challenging colleague? If so, how will you deal with that in a productive way and not take that home with you when your day ends? Is there a project due? How will you structure your time? You can do the same thing when you're taking a walk or working out. How far will you go? How much time do you have? What will keep you motivated?

Or your intentions can be as simple as making a list of things that are bugging you because they're not done yet, and identifying one small thing on the list that you *will* do that day. Make this task as small as you want: walking for twenty minutes, organizing a single shelf or drawer, or writing a tricky email you've been putting off. Then promise yourself you won't go to sleep till it's done, and honor yourself by keeping that promise. It's empowering, and it's a way to look forward to the day ahead. The other thing that happens when you keep your word to yourself is that other people will find you trustworthy too. And you'll notice that more trustworthy people enter your sphere. I swear by this truth.

By holding your intentions as you go through your day, you may find yourself drawing the people and circumstances that best suit you into your life, as if by magic. But it's not by magic: when you're aligned with your intentions, you attract what's true to you. First, you have to know what your intentions are, and then visualize and believe what or who you'd like to attract. I don't know of any situation where this approach doesn't help.

One of My Favorite Books

I'm a big fan of *Calling in "The One"* by Katherine Woodward Thomas. However, I'm *not* a big fan of the title or the artwork, and I've made this disclaimer to everyone I've given the book to! (As did my friend who first recommended it to me.)

Although it's marketed toward those who wish to find the love of their life, I feel that the true focus of the book is in helping you remove obstacles you've held onto your entire life—the past hurts and behaviors you've unintentionally absorbed that may be forcing you to repeat patterns until you finally learn from them. The "one" in the title is you. It stands to reason, of course, that you have the best chance of attracting the healthiest possible partner when you're the healthiest possible version of yourself. (I did meet someone who became one of my most significant friends while I was in the middle of working through the book—and many others immediately followed.) I believe the energy this book set in motion for me changed my life. It also coincided with my turning forty, which is a massive milestone anyway. Add to that the clearing away of old detritus that was no longer serving me, and forgiveness toward those I still had left to forgive, and it was a whole wide world of new.

These concepts reinforced what I'd already learned through years of experience: a lot of peace comes from simply working to the best of your abilities and not expecting that whomever you meet will be in your life forever. I'm not in touch with most of the countless people I've worked with on the hundred-plus jobs I've had over the years. I'd be happy to run into almost any of them (I can count the exceptions on one hand), but it's a rare experience when you find yourself connecting deeply with someone at work in a way that translates to developing a day-in-day-out, lifelong friendship.

Since completing *Calling in "The One,"* I've been much happier, more peaceful, and more aligned with attracting all that is leading me to my true purpose. The chapters are short and full of wisdom, and the deepest work is done by you, the reader. This involves a lot of intense journaling, writing letters to people in your past (whether you ever choose to send them is up to you), and things of that nature.

Let's Talk About Intuition

When I was in the process of moving—not quite in my new house yet, working in Vancouver—and people asked me where I lived, telling them *Nashville* rather than *LA* for the first time instantly made me feel more at home in my skin. That spoke volumes to my having made the right choice.

Listening to what feels true when you say it aloud is all about trusting your instincts and believing in the power of your intuition. Even before I'd officially moved into my new home, I loved sharing how excited Ernest had been when I first brought him to meet my prospective new house. He appeared to understand that I was bringing him to see if he wanted to live there, to see how he responded. When I let him go in the backyard, his spirit seemed to soar. He was racing around, like he couldn't believe there was all that space, and he was *so* happy. He gave it his unbridled paws up! In many ways, he's always been like a little mirror of me. And I couldn't have expressed my feelings better myself.

Intuition is often undervalued, I think, because it's not something you can quantify. We all experience it though—those moments when your gut says, *Do it!* or *Don't do it!* even when you can't explain why. These moments can lead to regret, if you didn't listen when something inside you was trying to get your attention.

As an actor, I now trust my intuition when it comes to whether to put myself on tape for an audition or not. I don't want to invest my time and my energy if my gut tells me I shouldn't be part of a project. When you're meeting new people, whether in person or by virtual means, you can often tell what your vibe together might be by the way your energy shifts, and whether your body feels peaceful and authentic.

On a different intuitive note, I've had the feeling that something was about to happen many times, and over the years, I find myself listening more and more when that sense arises. For instance, when I first laid eyes on Peter, who ended up becoming my first boyfriend, it was at the read-through he attended after he'd been cast to play my character's sister's husband on *Cybill*. I couldn't stop staring at him because I thought he was almost absurdly the complete embodiment of what I'd imagined my "ideal" to be at that time in my life, if I could have drawn him into existence.

I whispered something innocent to that effect in Dedee's ear (I think my exact words were, "Don't you think he's *so handsome?*"). She looked at me with delight, since she'd never heard me talk about any guy in that way before, and whispered back that although he wasn't *her* type—girl code to "go for it"—she thought it was fantastic that he was *my* type. I had that absolute *yes* feeling that if I were to date someone at that moment in time, that's who it would be. After almost a year of becoming friends and awkwardly flirting, we did date for three years.

A few years ago, I was doing a convention in Frankfurt, and a friend was going to be in Oslo and Stockholm right after that, so I decided to go visit. I'd never been to Scandinavia before, and something in me desperately wanted to go to Copenhagen. I couldn't figure out why, but a detour didn't quite make sense. I'd only have one day there, so I reluctantly opted to skip it. When I arrived at the airport for my flight to Oslo, they had a freak late-April snowstorm, and my flight got switched to Copenhagen after all. I was put up in a hotel and told I'd have about nineteen hours to spend in Denmark before my connecting flight.

At this point, I was absolutely convinced I was going to meet somebody, at the airport, or in some dark restaurant. Or we'd bump into one another on the street, like in a Hallmark Christmas movie. It would be the greatest love story of my life, and we never would have met if I hadn't gone to Copenhagen!

Well, nothing like that happened, and I didn't meaningfully converse with a single soul during my wanderings, but I walked all over the city in blissful solitude and had a wonderful and memorable time in Copenhagen. So, by that measure, I *was* meant to be there.

The Power of Journaling

Much like feeling that something is missing if I start my day without finding time to meditate, I love to finish my day with journaling. Even if it's only two minutes, right before I turn out the light, I relish spending that quiet time with my journal and handwriting for a few moments.

Journaling doesn't have to be a commitment to a book-length opus or to a "spill-all" diary. There's also no need to recount everything you did that day, from beginning to end. You don't need to turn it into a list of things you vow to do better tomorrow. It can be whatever *you* want it to be!

Why Journaling Is So Effective

When I was a teenager, I started writing in blue-lined paper notebooks every night. I was feeling powerless and wanting more than anything to find a way to get my thoughts out of my mind, as well as to try to better connect with God, and to figure out what that represented to me, since I'd never belonged to a specific religion. I would free-form write whatever was going on with me, almost like therapy, especially when something was really bothering me. Later, when I'd moved to LA, I would blurt out whatever I was thinking, but on my typewriter. I still have pages and pages of typewritten stream of consciousness from those years.

Doing this kind of purge-writing is powerful. It's helpful even if you don't intend to ever share it with anybody, or if you plan to burn what you wrote. Instead of saying what you need to say aloud, you're writing it out instead. You can then review what you wrote, and often, if you're looking for an answer to something, one will come to you. One way to think of this is to think of what you wrote as though a friend were sharing the dilemma you just poured out on the page. For example, if someone keeps disappointing you, you might recognize that the only thing that's going to change is you. Once you take on that responsibility, people who have been challenging in your life either vanish and you don't miss them as much as you thought you would, or they feel that energetic shift, and their behavior improves.

I've kept all of my journals, because they're a beautiful reflection of who I was at different times in my life. Rereading them brings everything back—all the people who were important to me, or people I thought I was madly in love with. It's a potent reminder that everything changes. We grow and we expand, and the way we react to certain outside forces changes and shifts as well. Thanks to my journaling, I've become a lot more peaceful and a much better observer of my own mind, so I can prevent little things that happened in my day from getting under my skin and causing me to feel imbalanced, perhaps without knowing why.

I don't always do my free-form, heavy duty journaling in my house, because I've found that anything that puts you slightly off-balance—such as leaving your comfort zone—can trigger all sorts of wonderful things. Going to different places can propel your mind in a direction it doesn't normally go. There's something great about going to a coffee shop, bar, or restaurant and sitting by yourself—like taking yourself on a date with your computer or notebook, to gather your ideas and get a clearer focus on what you want to deal with. Free-form journaling when you have no other distractions can be amazingly therapeutic.

Journaling also can help you manage the kind of anxiety that wakes you up in the middle of the night. When that happens to me, I grab my phone or my journal and start blurting out in written form what's on my mind. I've gotten some of my best writing done on my phone in the wee hours—some much-needed research, shopping, errand organizing, and of course, song lyrics. Once you solve that mental block or figure out what's irking you, or you just get up and take care of some things that are keeping you from resting, you'll not only feel incredibly productive but also sleep better afterward.

Most of the time, I use an actual journal instead of my laptop or phone, so I'm not distracted by an urge to check social media or the news. It's a small change to my routine, but it requires a serious commitment—though with big rewards. I like Moleskine journals because the paper is very smooth for writing on, and I always have a few on hand in case I'm about to run out of space. If you live in a household where you don't want your writing found, you can purchase journals with locks, or if you write on a computer, password protect your files. Journaling is about writing your most private and intimate thoughts, and unless you choose otherwise, they're for you and you alone.

> To be able to think back to what happened in this past day of your life, and realize how much was accomplished and how much happened that was good, is such a beautiful gift to yourself, and a testament to all the magic of just being alive.

Journaling About Gratitude

Journaling naturally helps you focus inward, and it can easily lead into meditation right before you go to sleep. If you're tired, it's more likely to make you feel sleepy too. Writing gives me a healthy closing routine for the day and, just as important, it allows me to practice gratitude.

Creating nightly gratitude lists has become one of my most empowering small changes. All you need to do is write down five things that happened that day that you're grateful for—even if it felt like the worst day ever. On such a day, if you go to bed without writing anything positive, the overriding feeling in your heart will be that the day sucked. Writing gratitude lists helps me to realize that often, just one particular thing bothered me or went wrong. Then it's up to me to either isolate that incident or let it affect the rest of the day, or even the next day or two. Besides, there's always *something* that happened during the day that I can remember being great—if only a beautiful smile I shared from across the street with a stranger and their sweet dog, or an especially delicious piece of food, or a plant or a bird. It may sound silly at first, but it makes a difference.

Good Morning to You!

As a complement to your nighttime journaling, try this. When you wake up, whether you're with a partner or on your own, I invite you to take a moment to say good morning to yourself. If you're like me, you have vivid dreams that can linger for a moment or two or longer. In those dreams, perhaps you're a child, teenager, or younger adult version of yourself. Whether you do dream, or wake up and need to get on with your day, take a moment to glance in a mirror and acknowledge the beautiful you in your reflection, fresh out of sleep. There's an innocence there, a freshness you'll see even if there are things about your appearance that aren't your favorites. Find something beautiful in that reflection, and I guarantee that when you see that beauty, others will too.

Over the years, I've been surprised to discover that, as I gather my thoughts at day's end, tracing back over the hours of it for beautiful occurrences, many of the wonderful little things that happened to me during the day were nearly forgotten, and would have been had I not committed them to paper. I'm often amazed by how full my day was. And then I fall asleep in that place of gratitude, and it sets the tone for more of these good things to come my way the next day. It gives me a great sense of peace. It also gives me more lucid and insightful dreams, and I hope your journaling will do that for you as well.

Another thing I love about gratitude lists is that they have a way of directing you back to what intentions you want to set for the next day, without you even meaning to. By reminding yourself about what happened that made you feel good that day, you're more likely to identify what will make you feel good the *next* day and become more mindful of those moments. You'll start noticing things you want to remember to write about later that night.

As I write this, I'm winding down for bed and thinking of a visit I had today with a friend I hadn't seen in a few years. When she was leaving, she said she'd been feeling this heaviness in her stomach—anxiety, concern over COVID-19 and the state of our country and our world, and wondering how we all go forward from here—and she noted that, having talked to me for those hours, the heaviness was lifted for the first time that she could remember in months. I'm tearing up while writing this. What an honor to hear that! It'll top this evening's gratitude list.

You can, of course, write your list lightning-fast if you're feeling uninspired or are very tired. But once you think of one thing, I bet you'll soon have a cavalcade of gratitude. If I'm feeling inspired, I frequently end up going into a reflective state and journal more than I intended to, because something I'm grateful for tumbles over into something I wish I'd handled differently or something that's bothering or perplexing me. Then I'm off on another tangent, and that's nice too. But I do always make a point of ending with gratitude—even if in that moment it's mostly for the work left to do and the questions raised, which an unsettling scenario can reveal.

A Sample Gratitude Journal Entry

Whether they seem mundane or profound, anything you write down is important!

My own gratitude journalings range from deep to trivial, and from long to extremely short. As I mentioned earlier, journals are for you and you alone, but here's a small one to share as an example, from while I was repairing my home after the tornado.

May 18, 2020

Grateful for the meeting with landscapers! I will have such a gorgeous backyard. I am flooded with joy! Grateful for another beautiful talk with XYZ, and to have inspired her to write gratitude tonight. Grateful for a day of decisions, choosing my floor finish. Finding ever more things to be improved at my home. Light and improvement everywhere! Grateful that XYZ reached out twice. And right after I nearly texted about owl, she texted, wanting to share about coyote. My heart is so full. Seeing possibility everywhere. Just happy.

PART IV

Caring for Your

body

CHAPTER 7

Love Your Body—and Watch It Transform

Nobody sees you when everyone's looking
Hiding in plain view
Sometimes you need to forget where you came from
To fall where you belong

—"CHASING SHADOWS"

Having a nutritious plant-based diet and a clear mind means that I'm more likely to take care of my body—and that means incorporating movement and exercise into my day-to-day routine. You don't have to live in the gym and be utterly obsessed with workouts to stay in pretty good shape. I know this because I live it!

But I didn't come to this knowledge easily. In fact, I went through years when I was a teenager and young adult keeping my unhealthy relationship with food a secret. It didn't help that I worked in a business where, particularly at that time, super-thin was the absolute standard for women. Now, thankfully, I've learned how to pay close attention to my triggers and love the body I'm in, in a way I once never thought possible.

Body Image, Amplified by a Life in Front of Cameras

The entertainment business, as far as it has come in terms of inclusivity and acceptance of all body shapes and types, is still one in which judging, regulating, and shaming people for their appearance is a daily reality. If you put yourself out there, you'll be on the receiving end of labeling and body-image scrutiny. Thankfully, as a society, I'd offer that we're becoming less tolerant of that, and rude comments by individuals or news outlets are often called out by the masses. Back when I started acting, though, I fully accepted that judgment on my appearance and needing to fit a mold were part of being an actor. I didn't recognize the ripple effects until much later.

After I'd taped the *Wheel of Fortune* Teen Week episode I mentioned in chapter 1, I watched the episode a few months later, back in Worcester, with my family. Someone remarked on how unusually thin they'd thought Vanna White had been in person, while on TV she just looked perfect. By comparison, it was said, on camera I looked heavier than I actually was—proving the old adage that "the camera puts on ten pounds," which was something I'd heard my whole life. Of course, I was *not* remotely heavy, and I didn't look heavy on camera either. I had never, until then, thought about my body shape or size. That all changed. I told myself I needed to lose weight. *Fast.*

I limited my caloric intake to 1,400 calories a day. If I was a few calories over the limit the previous day, I'd make up for it the next day by eating even less. I printed out calorie-breakdown lists and posted them on the kitchen wall. I measured precise portions. I ate my meals as slowly as I could, counting how many times I chewed each bite, and drank tons of water with them to make me feel fuller. My period stopped for a year.

By the time I moved back to LA in 1992, I was five feet nine and weighed only 110 pounds. I heard no more comments about the "baby fat" I'd had as a younger teen. In fact, several people said the opposite—that I'd look better with "a little meat on my bones."

As anyone who's struggled with eating issues would attest, the fear of being out of control that leads to anorexia can also swing the other direction, to using food to stuff away your feelings. By seventeen, I had the freedom of living in my first rented apartment on my own. Since I was underage, my dad agreed to cosign the lease for me, in a demonstration of love and faith in me that still feels as present as the day I called him from a pay phone on a street corner in Westwood to ask him to. Playing piano to pay my rent and bills made me an atypical teen, when most kids my age would have been thinking about high school graduation. But, like many teenagers, unusual upbringing or not, I felt very grown-up on the outside and very lonely on the inside.

David Lynch cast me once again, in a magnificent (and grown-up—including my first ever kiss, on- or off-screen!) role opposite Crispin Glover in the HBO movie *Hotel Room*, and I had a small but noticeable part in a film called *Bodies, Rest & Motion* that garnered me some attention. After a lengthy audition process and a full-day mix and match with the entire cast, I was offered a role in the iconic high school film *Dazed and Confused*. But my agents lost the deal by refusing to agree to the contract, which would sign me up for two potential sequels, something I learned of only when they told me the offer had been rescinded. (Like sequels would have been a bad thing at that stage? I found new representation promptly after that.)

I can see, looking back, I was being given all the signs that, yes, I was in the right place, I was supposed to be acting, and I needed to keep doing good work and have faith I'd find my way. But the fact of it was, I was going on multiple auditions a day (as I mentioned in chapter 1), sitting in waiting rooms with girls who looked like they all would have been homecoming queen, and my ratio of auditions to actual jobs felt disheartening. I started to become fearful that I wouldn't get enough acting work to make a living, and the people back home who said, "You'll be back" were right, and that I wasn't pretty enough or good enough.

I started to lead a bizarre double life in which I'd parrot my old dietary restrictions while out, then binge when I came home (still sticking to the restrictions in the beginning—just eating way too much). The more I ate, the worse I felt about myself, so the more I would eat. I'd dine out with new friends and order unsalted, steamed vegetables and some plain grilled chicken. Then I'd go home and scarf down a jar of unsalted almond butter, a loaf of unrefined bread, and a bag of peaches or cherries. In one night.

Between the ages of sixteen and nineteen, I gained forty-five pounds. Since I'm tall, it wasn't as obvious that I had a problem with disordered eating as it might have been if I were smaller—my frame is petite, but my height meant I could distribute the weight well and everyone assumed it was still that baby fat I'd once had. The truth is, I was nowhere near "heavy." And most importantly, I can see now that I looked beautiful.

At seventeen, one of my favorite audition outfits was a long-sleeved, button-down black blouse that I tied at the waist and paired with jeans. The jeans had kind of a mid-rise waist, and you could see my belly. One day, my then-manager called and said several of the casting directors had told her that if I was going to wear tops like that I should do more sit-ups or be thinner. My manager was a middle-aged woman who was in a position to nurture, yet she honestly thought that sharing this feedback was doing me a favor, so I'd get more jobs.

This was reinforced a few weeks later, when I did a headshot shoot with a fashion photographer. When we were looking at the proof sheets, he said, "You know, you'd be a knockout if you lost fifteen pounds. You could model." He meant it as a compliment, but instead of thinking, *Okay, I'm going to lose fifteen pounds and be a knockout and model*, I thought, *He's right. I'm not pretty enough. I'm too heavy. Everyone can see it.*

Comments like these were the voices in my head as I kept binging with a vengeance. Yet the weight wasn't what was stopping me from reaching my potential—it was the other issues, the ones that led to the unhealthy eating habits in the first place, which were holding me back from being present and doing the best work I could. I cringe to remember several huge auditions where I knew I was the first choice yet spent the night before binge eating, avoiding working on my scenes. Being told that I was heavier than optimal meant that if I didn't get the roles I dreamed of, if I couldn't quite make it, at least the (perceived) reason for my rejection was in my control. But I didn't do my best work *because* I'd been self-sabotaging. I have no doubt this is why I didn't get those early jobs.

The summer before I turned eighteen, I was invited to participate in the Sundance Institute summer lab. It was a two-week gathering where up-and-coming filmmakers were awarded the opportunity to workshop their projects with established directors, crew, and professional/experienced actors (I know—a big honor to be asked, and another sign I was making an impression). I was by far the youngest one there—the rest of the younger actors were in their mid-twenties—and everyone was kind enough to take me under their wing. I joined them when they went out in nearby Provo, and they smuggled me into bars where I sipped water and juice and tried to fit in. Then we'd go out to eat and I'd have my steamed vegetables like the good girl I thought that made me, but back at the house I'd get up in the middle of the night and stuff myself with what I'd bought at the grocery store—an innocent-seeming (and incredibly weird) combo of frozen corn kernels, milk, and cereal, mixed together. Regardless of what you're eating, it doesn't take an expert to see something's not right when you're sitting in a darkened kitchen, silently stuffing yourself in the wee hours.

One day when we were done working, the topic of where to go to eat came up, and someone questioned whether there'd be something I *could* eat there. The actor Priscilla Pointer (whose daughter Amy Irving was also there;

Priscilla was best-known for playing Amy's mother in the movie *Carrie*), turned toward me with a scowl. "*Why* do you eat like that?" she asked.

"It's how I've always eaten," I replied, startled.

"You don't need to," she said bluntly. "It makes you seem strange."

I found myself halfheartedly explaining my lifelong rules, and that eating this way was better for me. "No one else has ever said they had a problem with the way I eat," I added defensively.

Priscilla's voice softened a bit. "Well, maybe no one ever cared enough to tell you before," she said, then left the room. I dismissed her comments because I wasn't yet able to be receptive to them. Later, I realized it was a defining moment.

The next spring, working on *Mr. Holland's Opus*, during the shoot I'd eat my saltless, steamed cuisine on set and on nights out with the crew. Then going back to my room, I'd order Häagen-Dazs ice cream sundaes (by now having tasted chocolate and sugar), answering the door for room service the instant they arrived, hoping no one from the production would be walking by. Then I'd set my alarm and walk to the nearest grocery store at 7:00 a.m., thinking the likelihood of running into anyone from the movie at that time was pretty slim. I'd stock my cart with Pepperidge Farms cookies, croissants, and the most sugary granolas I could find. If I'd been found out, what did I think they would think? I have honestly no idea. I was so used to not eating normally—and it was so ingrained in me that I was "different" in that way—I couldn't imagine *not* having that distinction. It may sound incredible, but it was as much a part of my identity as the fact that I was a redhead.

Fortunately, a warm-hearted producer, whose daughter was only a few years younger, somehow intuited that I needed guidance. I was referred to a wonderful therapist in LA who specialized in treating eating disorders. This was the beginning of many, many small changes—not only in how I approached food but also in the revelation that there is no quick-fix answer to anything.

I realized that food is the most pervasive addiction there is because, unlike other substances, you cannot do without it or give it up cold turkey. While my struggles with food didn't end at eighteen, when I started working intensely with my first therapist, the acknowledgment of my issues began there—and so did the healing. I was given strategies so that I wouldn't succumb to bingeing every time I wanted to. One simple but effective one was this: she asked how much I'd normally spend on one of these late-night grocery store haunts. I came up with twenty dollars, which went a long way in 1994 and was a lot to spend at a time when money was tight for me. She suggested that the next time I felt the urge, I should take a twenty-dollar bill, tear it into shreds, and flush it down the toilet.

When I was cast on *Cybill*, my existing body size was a defining part of who Zoey was and an asset in helping me to land the role. While some of the reviews mentioned how refreshingly "normal" my body was, the word *zaftig* was thrown around more than once, from makeup artists and publicists and critics. Regardless of whether that was meant as a compliment, as I'm sure you can guess already, I didn't take it as such. Thank goodness I was working with my therapist and had gotten beyond the first step in recovery to where I was no longer hiding my struggles with food. I was making real friends, and I now was being recognized on a daily basis for the first time ever. Admittedly, this was exactly what I'd been wanting—proof, again, that I was in the right world and could make a career out of acting and have a blast doing it.

At the same time, though, I took *zaftig* as a challenge to lose those fifteen pounds and be the knockout that photographer had promised I'd be, only this time with the eyes of an international audience upon me. Once filming our first season finished, I took dietary supplements my publicist had recommended, including the stimulant ma huang (which we now know can dangerously increase your heart rate but was all the rage at the time), the allegedly fat-burning chromium picolinate, and followed a diet consisting of four small meals a day: protein and a lean vegetable. I also ran six miles, twice around the Lake Hollywood reservoir jogging path, nearly every day. I quickly dropped about twenty pounds and was thrilled to show up to my first wardrobe fitting for season two several sizes smaller—which in turn meant I was now fitting into skinny jeans and tight-fitting tops. I also took the hair and makeup team up on their offer to spruce up my look to go along with my new clothes. These changes were never mentioned on the show—I just suddenly had masses of long ringlets and flawless eye makeup instead of the straight, messy hair/grungy teenager look I'd had only a few months earlier. When a letter appeared in *USA Today*'s Life section, inquiring if a different actress was now playing Zoey, I couldn't have been more proud. My publicist called to tell me they were asking for a comment, and I remember the quote they used: "Alicia Witt is thrilled you noticed her new look!"

The show was such a hit that after only its first season, it was nominated for a Golden Globe for best comedy series, as well as nods for Cybill Shepherd and Christine Baranski. By the time of the Golden Globe ceremony in January 1996, I had my gown and jewelry picked out, and hair and makeup artists due to arrive early that afternoon to get me ready. It was especially exciting because the Globes were the only ceremony at that time, besides the SAG Awards, where if the show won, the entire cast went up on stage. But the anxiety of appearing before all those cameras, feeling I'd already gained some weight back, and worrying I'd look *zaftig* in my gown, all manifested in me stuffing myself in front of the TV the night before with multiple pints of ice cream, along with other things I'd neglected to properly store in the fridge. I woke up at 5:00 a.m., horribly sick. After hours of throwing up too many times to count and not being able to keep down any water, I knew I was in danger of dehydration or worse, so I called a taxi to take me to the Cedars-Sinai emergency room.

A couple of bags of IV fluid later, I was ready to go home to finish my recovery, just in time to see my friends walk the red carpet at the pre-Globes event, and then the awards themselves. Sure enough, we won! I was sitting on my living room floor, watching alone as all my castmates and the writers and producers took the stage triumphantly. My eyes drifted over to that beautiful black dress hanging on the back of my bedroom door, unworn. Although I was still a few years away from learning my lesson for good, the seeds were planted just a bit deeper that night.

To date, this is the only show I've been involved with that has won best series at the Golden Globes. I didn't share that I'd binged the night before with *anyone*—I was too embarrassed—but deep down, I knew there had to be a better answer than stuffing my feelings away. All the anxiety I had felt melted away into the clarity of how silly it had been, and I only wished I could have been there, celebrating with my friends. If I had a do-over, I'd choose to have taken a hot bath, journaled some, and gone to bed early in anticipation of the exciting day ahead. Who knows? Maybe it was a stomach flu, and I would've woken up sick anyway.

But my gut told me it was a lesson I was supposed to learn. (Um, no pun intended?)

Slowly, my need to binge lessened. I wasn't spending a lot of time on my own, stuffing myself with food anymore. I was busy with work, and shortly after this, I was in my first relationship.

Fast-forward to my starring role in the 1998 thriller *Urban Legend*. We shot it on the outskirts of Toronto in April. Five full weeks of the schedule were night shoots, with me running through the rain for what felt like about a quarter of the movie, warning everyone about a serial killer on the loose. The rain was scripted, so even if it wasn't raining for real (which it was, a lot of the time), a rain machine was propped on a crane, ensuring the requisite water continued to fall from the skies above. If I wasn't physically in the rain in a scene, my character had just come in from the rain, which meant I had to be hosed down from head to foot before entering an indoor scene. I was dripping wet and freezing cold, and since I wasn't yet vegan, I was wearing a suede jacket and high-heeled leather boots and blue jeans, which absorbed all the water and made me even colder. I couldn't get warm.

We'd have "lunch" at 12:30 a.m. and wrap at 6:30 a.m. I'd go home, and instead of going to bed, I'd eat something heavy, like pasta, to put myself into a food coma because I was still wired and stressed. It was hard work, physically and emotionally, and I was in almost every scene. As they say in the horror genre, I was the "final girl," aka the last one alive.

I gained weight while filming, which you can see in the movie, which made me feel less and less pretty, and therefore less and less confident. And as we've already established, this creates a loop: the less confident I felt, the more I ate.

One day about midway through the shoot, the lone female producer came into my trailer and approached me like, *We've got to stick together because we're the girls on this shoot.* Just as I was thinking how nice it was that she wanted to be friends, she said, "I wanted to say that sometimes padded bras are really great because they just give you a nice shape under sweaters and things. And, um, you know . . . *I* wear a padded bra!" The "girl talk" ended abruptly after I responded less than enthusiastically to this suggestion, so I deduced that she'd been sent in there to ask me to wear a padded bra to make my breasts look bigger under my sweater. They didn't tell me to lose weight. But perhaps the idea was: If I was going to be heavier, then why not make my breasts bigger too?

By the time I appeared on *The Sopranos* a year and a half later, playing the titular "D-Girl" in season two, I was twenty-four, slender, and womanly, just in time for my first sex scene (with Michael Imperioli, who played Christopher). This was my first TV role with major visibility after my run on *Cybill*, and the perception was that I'd suddenly grown up and transformed into a sexy young woman. Consequently, I got a lot of attention. I ended up on the cover of *Stuff*, a men's magazine of the day, in February 2000, with the tagline "Red Hot!" I was wearing a crop top that had fallen back over my shoulders, a leopard-print bra, and a miniscule bikini bottom. And my now-tiny belly was on full display.

People looked at that photo (and still remark on my body in that sex scene) and thought I was the hottest I've ever been. They didn't know I was so thin because within that past year I'd discovered bulimia as a way of stuffing myself when I felt lonely—but without gaining the weight. I'd never been bulimic before, but I remember trying it for the first time in a hotel room, on location where I'd just arrived to film a movie. I thought I'd found some magic trick. From 1999 through mid-2000, I was out of control. It breaks my heart to remember that.

I got so ill from my bulimia that one night at my new house in LA, I thought I was having a heart attack because my heart was beating so fast. In that moment, I swore on my dog Jake's life that I would never purge again. I never did—and I never will. No slimness is worth it, and the truth is, after purging for a year, your body is so utterly messed up that you can't digest food properly, your metabolism is destroyed, and you gain weight when you eat even a tiny meal. It's awful in every way.

As with any addictive behavior, you are the only one who can make the ultimate choice to stop. I continued to work with therapists over the years, and with them I've had many experiences that have changed my life and helped me to grow exponentially. Over the years, the focus of this work has often been the demise of a relationship that broke my heart, or trying to ensure I engage in healthy behavior while being in a relationship, or sorting through something I was aware I could use some help with.

The beautiful thing about therapy is that as you learn and change, the therapy you need—and the therapist who's right for you—can also change. It also bears sharing that, when I was bulimic, I didn't actually *want* to change. I was embarrassed, but I also liked the way my body looked. When I got back into therapy shortly after my conversation with God, in which I agreed to never purge again, I was addressing the feelings of insecurity and desperation that led me to abuse my body in that way. For instance, that therapist helped me accept the end of a relationship a few months later with a charismatic man I thought I was deeply in love with, despite him treating me in ways I should never have settled for. Therapy helped me to eventually work my way through those feelings and to fall in love with a very good man who became my longest relationship.

One cornerstone of my eating disorder was that, night after night, I'd say, "This is the last time," and then devour a high-calorie meal. Then the next night I'd say the same thing, when what I should have been saying was, "I want a little bit of this because it tastes good. Tomorrow I might have a little more. I don't have to eat it all tonight until I'm about to explode." This is easier said than done when you're in the throes of something, but it works long-term. It's something I work on still to this day.

I've learned to embrace the feeling of being satiated but not stuffed. I've also learned there are practical ways of feeling full without packing on the calories, which is especially important as you grow older and need to pay even more attention to excess weight. Eating too many simple carbohydrates in the form of grains—like a bagel or a donut, for example—will cause your blood sugar to spike and leave you hungry again an hour later, so it's better to fill up on complex carbs such as beans, fresh vegetables and fruits, and whole grains in moderation. I still love coconut or oat or cashew ice cream, but certain foods, like those, are my Achilles' heel and could lead to my eating too much of them. So I either resist the urge to buy them, or I scoop my serving into a bowl and make myself a cup of tea or have a big glass of water half an hour later, if I feel I'm craving more of it than I need. And sometimes I do eat the whole pint! But my body is balanced enough now that if I do, I'll be less hungry the next day, and I'll not likely want to do that again for a while.

One benefit of becoming more of an experienced actor (in credits as well as age) is that nobody would dare tell me to lose weight or wear a padded bra anymore. I can't remember the last time I've stepped on a scale . . . well, yes I can. It's at my yearly physical or when I have a cast checkup before filming a movie. I couldn't care less what I weigh. And the less I think about it and simply listen to my body, the more effortless it is to maintain my weight. I rarely put on a pair of jeans and think, *Wow, those are getting snug!* And if I do—or if I am observing my tummy feeling a tad more cushioned than it normally is, between acting jobs—I pay more attention to being diligent with my workout routine for the next few weeks or make my portions a bit smaller. (They're generally huge, as we've established!) The small changes I've made across all areas of my life make me feel happy, confident, and healthy—and comfortable in my own skin.

The Benefits of Yoga

You can read all about the importance of exercise in chapter 10, but one important practice that has helped me learn to love my body is yoga. It has amazing benefits—not only the flexibility and strength it gives me, but the controlled breathing to bring calm and undo stress.

I discovered yoga through my friend Caroline, a writer who used to live in LA. She suggested that I accompany her to the now-gone Maha Yoga, which had a ridiculously popular class that was almost a cross between aerobics and slow yoga. It was very fast-paced, very crowded, very sweaty, and also sometimes very strange, being packed like sardines into the room, with mats placed end to end during particularly crowded classes. But everyone accepted that as part of the deal, and it was worth it. The music was loud and pulsing, and before you knew it, you'd be covered in sweat from an incredibly good workout as the ninety minutes flew right by. What was fun for me as a beginner was to watch what other people were doing and approximate it, and then the instructor would weave through the throngs of mats and make adjustments before we cooled down with a lot of stretching.

Other instructors at Maha were much more traditional and had less crowded classes, so I was able to learn more of the basics, in part because they were able to do more hands-on corrections. I realized how helpful it is to take classes and get the proper positions programmed into your muscle memory so you can then practice on your own. When an instructor adjusts your pose a bit, and you feel those little muscles engage and realize what the position is supposed to be doing for you, it's a beautiful thing.

One instructor, Ish Moran, was the coolest guy—a correctional officer who taught yoga on the side! I had assumed he was in his early forties because looking at him, there was no conceivable way that he could be any older than that. When he told me, nonchalantly, that he was sixty-five, I just about had to pick my jaw off the floor. What living proof of how wonderful yoga is—not just for mental clarity and physical strength, but for your appearance, especially as you age! Yoga uses your own body weight to strengthen and lengthen your muscles and add flexibility to your joints. I think of yoga as a combination of Pilates and weightlifting and meditation all rolled into one.

As my dad once observed when he was visiting me and asked how my day was, "You always say you've had a really good day when it's a day you've done yoga." I've never forgotten that! Now I do my best to try to fit in at least a fifteen-minute session when I don't have time to go to a class, because I want to have that "good day" feeling every day.

De-stress with Yoga Breathing

The breathing techniques yoga teaches you can be incredibly helpful in times of stress. I do a few rounds of this routine if I'm about to go on stage to speak or to perform, and my heart is beating so fast from butterflies that I know I need to center myself. I've also done this breathing in other difficult moments, particularly if I'm about to have a conversation with someone that might be challenging or makes me feel nervous.

The process of connecting your breath to the movements adjusts your mood and your breathing and helps connect you back into your body.

1. From a standing position, bend down and hang your head and your arms, straight down to your feet. Keep your legs straight as well.
2. Come up on your fingertips with a flat back, breathe in deeply, then exhale back down.
3. Rise up as you bring your arms straight up over your head.
4. Exhale, bring your hands to prayer position at your chest.
5. Inhale, bring your arms back up above your head.
6. Exhale, swan dive forward, and bend at the waist, back down toward your feet.

CHAPTER 8

Small Changes to Your Lifestyle

I saw your face change
Some kind of magic took a breath beneath your skin

—"FACE CHANGE"

Once you start incorporating a few small changes into your lifestyle, it becomes contagious!

I love talking about lifestyle topics with the people I meet, especially skincare and sun protection. Taking the best care of yourself will also lighten your budget; once you discover effective skincare products, you won't be endlessly trying new ones that never seem to work.

Getting Older—And Loving It

As you read in the previous chapter, the seemingly omnipresent suggestion that ultra-thin is the most desirable state of being can lead to eating disorders and despair. The demand for an eternally youthful face can be just as damaging.

In the entertainment biz, when people know how old you are, they see you as that age no matter what you look like. Hence, many people lie about their age. In my mid-twenties, I was sometimes told I was *too old* for certain roles I knew I was right for, simply because my age has always been accurate, given how young I was when I started acting. It used to frustrate me, especially when I'd research my peers who claimed to be eight years younger than they were, and they were being considered for a role I was closer to the right age for.

So one day I thought I'd subtract a couple of years from my age on IMDB—only two years, because I knew I couldn't get away with more than that. Within twenty-four hours, people were posting on the message board and referencing a *Good Housekeeping* magazine article from when I was two years old in 1977, so I couldn't have been *born* in 1977. End of experiment! I realized my age wasn't something I'd ever have the choice to lie about, and I'm glad about that anyway. I'm happy to go out into the world and tell everyone how old I am, because I'm proud of how I've taken care of myself over the years—but I also think our age is a blessing and gift!

A few actors I can think of are exactly my age, such as Drew Barrymore, Kate Winslet, and Angelina Jolie, as well as my fellow Hallmark Christmas alumni Danica McKellar and Candace Cameron Bure. Then there are many others I've worked with over the last decade whose "official" ages are *definitely* not accurate. And it's not just women! I briefly joined the dating app Raya, out of curiosity to see if that was an interesting way to meet someone, and an actor ex of mine popped up. He's two months older than me—or perhaps I should say, he used to be. He's now five years younger, apparently!

Professional Scrutiny Leads to Professional Treatments

Not long ago, face-lifts or chemicals peels were the only treatments available that could tighten skin and remove wrinkles. Now, of course, there are dozens of much safer and less costly alternatives like injectable fillers, laser treatments, and infrared devices to help people minimize the signs of aging. This is great when you want to smooth out a few deep wrinkles or tone a few sags, and the work you can get done is often so subtle that you still look exactly like yourself, only rested and refreshed. This is *not* great, however, when people who are no longer in their twenties are expected to look as if they still are. This has led many performers and public figures to end up looking fake and plastic (and/or to only post photos with so many filters on them, it's impossible to tell what they really look like!). And the scary by-product of that, as I see it, is that nonpublic figures look at them and might think, *Oh, that's what beauty looks like these days.* I hate seeing my non-industry and industry friends alike getting more and more immobile in their beautiful faces. That's not beautiful to me.

Because my appearance has been something that, unavoidably, has been scrutinized as part of my lifelong chosen professional career(s), I'd never judge anyone who feels there's something about their face that no longer looks like what they believe they should look like. It's easy enough to try something like Botox, which wears off in a few months; if you aren't happy with the results, they'll fade away.

I've always been most drawn to faces that show expression and history—so for me (as of now!) Botox is not something I've felt compelled to try. I look to actors like Judi Dench and Maggie Smith as role models for the way I'd like to look when I'm in my eighties. Acting is all about letting every emotion show on your face, yet some actors (who are extremely successful) have such unnaturally smooth faces that I find it hard to focus on anything else when their foreheads aren't moving! Seeing that takes me right out of the performance, which upends my enjoyment of whatever I'm watching. It alarms me when I see how common it is these days for female actors to have their faces injected to the point where the only feature that reveals emotion is their eyes. (I know they're the window to the soul, but . . . c'mon!) It's even more jarring when the era is supposed to be the '50s or the '70s or the '90s . . . or you're in an apocalypse fighting for survival, but your face doesn't move? I deeply wish there were a way to reverse the accepted (and seemingly expected) "expressionless" standard of beauty. Why are personality-defining lines and proof of your time here on earth something to be erased?

Sometimes I wonder if I'm out of touch. But then I think perhaps this is merely a phase our society is going through. And I also want to say this: life is short. If *anything* about your appearance truly bothers you, if you can afford a treatment or procedure and you feel it will give you the results you seek, after researching it thoroughly, *go for it*. It's incredible that we live in a time when this is an option. But it breaks my heart when I see people going down a rabbit hole where you "fix" one thing, then something else looks older in comparison, and you have to "fix" that too. Then your face doesn't move anymore, and you think that looks ideal. For whatever it's worth, please know that I don't think that's ideal. Unique faces are interesting, appealing, and sexy.

I also wish there wasn't such a shroud of secrecy around cosmetic work. To that end, I'm proud to share my experience. In my mid-thirties, I developed under-eye bags that became more and more pronounced. They had nothing to do with how much sleep I got or if I drank too much or ate too much salt. They were genetic; my parents both have them. I'd do juice cleanses and not have any alcohol for two weeks as a test, and there was no effect whatsoever. I looked tired and sluggish all the time, even when I wasn't. I mean, I'm fine with looking fifty when I'm actually fifty, but looking fifty when I was forty was a different story! I'd tried to take such good care of my skin over the years, and in every other way, I felt it reflected that.

Even so, the roles I was starting to be considered for were all scripted older than I was (and I'm grateful, because some of those roles I played were life-changing; however, I definitely didn't want to *not* be considered for roles my age any longer). It was also becoming harder to do my makeup and to light me. No topical product, no cooling under-eye pads or de-puffer wand or Preparation H (yes, that's used sometimes) worked after a while. And under-eye bags do nothing to help you express yourself. If anything, they make it harder to see your eyes.

I researched what could be done and learned that the only remedy was a short, outpatient surgical procedure called a blepharoplasty.

After getting recommendations from my dermatologist, I booked the procedure with a highly regarded plastic surgeon whose entire practice is eyelid surgery. In the months leading up to it, I was wishing I could talk to, or read a testimonial from, someone in my business who'd had it done and could confirm I was making the right decision.

Many years earlier, on my first day of work on a series with a male actor, we were standing next to each other when the makeup artist came in to do final touches. As he worked under the actor's eyes with his sponge, moving the makeup around to get it perfect for the camera, I noticed for the first time that there were big bruises under the actor's eyes. "Oh my God, what happened?" I blurted (I thought he'd been in a fight). He glared daggers at me, and I instantly knew he'd had that surgery. I suddenly remembered that he'd had large bags under his eyes at the table read we'd done a few weeks earlier. As I quickly looked away, I wished he'd had a different reaction, because he looked fantastic. It *should* be empowering to share that you've had work done, especially when the results are amazing. The more people talk about plastic surgery or cosmetic dermatology, the less taboo it is to talk about it.

Right up until two days before the surgery, I was still trying to talk myself out of it. I was scared something would go wrong or that it would look strange or obvious. That weekend, I arrived in Charlotte to appear at a *Walking Dead* convention. After a light dinner and excellent night's sleep, the next morning I woke up and caught a glance at myself in the bathroom mirror, and burst out laughing. I looked like I hadn't slept in days, as well as dehydrated, hungover, and drunk at the same time—just *unhealthy*—when none of that was true, and I felt as fresh as a daisy. This was a good reminder of why I'd decided to have the procedure. I texted a snapshot of my "before" look to my best friends, so they could text it back to me in case I had cold feet the morning of! (I didn't. And I am so glad I went through with it.)

When I was twenty-three, I had a bump removed from the bridge of my nose. This bump first appeared when I was about nineteen years old, and over the next four years, it became more and more prominent. I was a klutzy young adult, constantly having freak accidents, walking into things, tripping over my own two feet as I entered a room. It seemed likely I'd gotten hit in the nose with something, probably a softball from my time playing on the *Cybill* softball league. (We were ranked dead last among all twenty-two teams representing the four major networks at the time, so it says a lot that I was by far the worst player on our team!) That was the opinion of the two doctors I saw for consultation, who said I didn't need a full nose job, where your nose has to be broken and reset. I didn't want a different nose, but I did want it to look like what it had before.

When I finally had the procedure, after filming *Urban Legend* but before its premiere, I was thrilled with the results. The only way I can describe it is that I looked on the outside like I *felt* I looked, if that makes sense. To me, the bump didn't look like me, because it hadn't always been there. After all the times I'd agonized over whether I should or shouldn't, I still have a vivid memory, as I was fading off under the light general anesthetic, of Christina Aguilera's "Reflection" playing.

Aside from those two procedures, I get laser facials regularly, which involve heat being applied to your upper layers of skin to stimulate collagen growth. I haven't had any fillers or injectables, which doesn't feel right for me, at least right now. I'm hopeful I can age as naturally as possible, while maintaining a face that's fun to look at, feels like me, and doesn't seem like someone whose main objective is appear as young as possible. I treasure my friends of all ages, and as beautiful as twenty-five-year-olds can be, it's growing older that makes us even more beautiful. And so much of this comes from the inside.

Tape It Up!

About twelve years ago, I was hired for a photo campaign for the lovely jewelry designed by Lisa Hoffman, who's married to Dustin, and his makeup artist came to do my face. In passing, she mentioned she was in her early fifties, and while she was working on me, I was transfixed by her beautiful skin, particularly her forehead. It was obvious she hadn't had any fillers, as she had some fine lines reflecting the life she'd lived, but her relaxed expression and natural beauty were stunning—exactly how I hoped to look at that age. I asked her how she managed not to have a frown line, and she said, "Do you want to know my secret? Right before I go to sleep, I use Scotch Tape on my forehead. I just put one strip on each side of the frown part and pull it toward my temples." She smiled. "I've been doing it for twenty years."

I love this tip because it came from a makeup professional who knew what she was doing—and I could see the results. I've tried it and it *does* work. But beware! One night I put the Scotch Tape on *after* I'd already applied my prescription Retin-A, and I also ripped it off way too quickly the next morning and in the opposite direction I'd applied it. Big mistake. For a few days I had what looked like tread marks on my forehead.

Be sure your forehead is clean and dry, or if you've applied a moisturizer, make sure it's absorbed and you've patted away any excess or oils before putting the tape on. When removing the tape, peel slowly and carefully, backward from how you applied it. If you do this even two nights in a row, I think you'll see the difference! It's also a great trick if you have a big event coming up that you're wanting to look extra-relaxed for.

My Skincare Routine

The way I eat and nourish my body is reflected in my skin. When I transitioned from a pescatarian diet to a nearly 100 percent plant-based one, I didn't recognize how much I was changing physically until it had already happened. For example, when I decided to stop eating dairy, within a month people started asking me what I was doing differently. I had already noticed that I felt less "heavy" in my body and that I was less congested in my throat—important for someone who uses her voice so much, in acting and in singing. But then my friends and colleagues started saying, "Wow, Alicia, you look so much younger! What are you doing to your skin? There's such a *clarity* to it."

I simply thought I was having good skin days . . . weeks and weeks of them!

In addition to my vegan diet, I've always had to pay attention to my skincare because I'm fair-skinned and burn easily. Sun exposure is the number one cause of skin damage, not to mention the obvious risk of melanoma, so I'm lucky I started wearing hats and sunscreen decades ago, which prevented some wrinkles that otherwise would have appeared by now. It's never too late to start using high-quality sunscreen, but not all sunscreens are alike. (More on this below!)

I don't use any skincare products, hair care products, or makeup that are tested on animals. One exception is prescription-strength retinol, which, because it's a pharmaceutical, was legally required to be tested on animals prior to being approved. Hopefully, one day the industry will catch up with the science, and animal testing will no longer be automatically required for pharmaceuticals. And truly, there's no longer a need anymore, as there are now electronically generated means of testing for allergies and reactions that simulate a human reaction with better accuracy than testing on animals. Fortunately, most beauty companies have listened to consumers, and animal testing is no longer the norm. You have many great products to choose from, but you still need to be a smart shopper and always read the labels if it's important to you to avoid animal cruelty in skincare.

Because my skin is well taken care of from the inside out, I have a basic skincare routine for the outside in. No matter your skin type, I think some version of this might help you too. At this point, if I skip my routine once in a while, it's not going to be the end of the world—but my skin will rebel if I skip for more than one night. It's much easier to prevent zits from forming than to get rid of them! And a small change I've needed to make is acknowledging that it's a simple thing to do, to apply your skincare routine no matter how tired or distracted or busy you might feel.

Wash Your Face

At night, I try to always wash my face with a warm, wet facecloth, along with a gentle liquid cleanser if I have makeup on. I like Arcona cleansers because they clean thoroughly, don't leave a residue, and can easily be rinsed off. Their products are almost entirely organically derived, smell incredible, and really do work. There is also an Ole Henriksen foaming cleanser that is gentle and does the trick. Desert Essence Thoroughly Clean Tea Tree Oily Face Wash cleanser is a cheap one for when your skin feels especially oily. It's also great for shoulders and back or anywhere that might need a little extra astringent.

Every other morning, I use Arcona Golden Grain Gommage as a refreshing start. This is best used in the shower since it has gentle exfoliating bits that are harder to remove with a facecloth. Another good, less costly alternative to this is Thrive Natural Face Scrub. I also believe in using a fresh facecloth every day. I know that may seem either obvious to some or overkill to others. But if you do your laundry once a week, you only need seven washcloths! I don't think it's a good idea to introduce yesterday's bacteria to your skin, even if you've rinsed the cloth and let it air dry. It's fine to reuse between morning and night; just use different sides.

If I'm at work and need to wear a lot of heavy makeup, or if I'm out and about with makeup on, the best beauty hack I've learned in the last couple of years is to take off all my foundation/powder in the T-zone and under my eyes every six to eight hours. Then you reapply whatever moisturizer and serum you like to use, let that soak in, and reapply your foundation to those areas.

I'd never suggest taking off eye makeup in the middle of your day, but if you bring some moist makeup removers to work (I like Arcona's cleansing pads), or wash your face before going out to dinner after a long day at work, that can go a huge distance in stopping breakouts before they happen, since you won't be clogging your pores by applying more makeup. Even if you don't wear a ton of foundation, it can be super helpful to cleanse off the grime your skin has built up during the day.

I've been doing this recently on all my jobs, but regardless of what you do for a living, it's great for anyone who wears makeup. It only takes a few minutes at most, and it's *so* worth it! Your skin will look much fresher. Of course, it's great for absolutely anyone who doesn't wear makeup too, including men. Sunscreen and moisturizer work best when they're reapplied regularly, and even the best products will start to block your pores if you reapply them on top of the oil your skin has naturally built up. I highly recommend taking two minutes at lunchtime to quickly wipe at least the T-zone off, and reapply your cream. Especially if you have problem skin, this will make a huge difference, for little time spent.

Don't Forget the Wipes!

Another absolute must for me is baby wipes. This isn't TMI—I'm serious! I think they're a game changer to have handy for whenever you visit the facilities. They're also invaluable in the battle many women have with UTIs, which are caused by bacteria that wipes can help fight. For only a few dollars a pack, you can't ask for a cheaper and more valuable preventative product. I'm always amazed at the number of adults I meet on a weekly basis who don't use them. I have some in my purse at all times, and if I forget to pack them in my suitcase, they're on my list of must-have items whenever I land in a new city, even for a few days. I like Seventh Generation because they're gentle, eco-friendly, and don't sting your sensitive parts.

Just remember that even if the wipes claim to be flushable, don't flush them—they clog the plumbing and contribute to fatbergs in the sewage system and harm ocean creatures as well. I know this isn't the most eco-friendly option available—but I'll be honest: I'd call this a situation where the benefit outweighs the harm. Try and cut down on your plastics use, and splurge on a couple of baby wipes a day, responsibly disposed of in the trash.

Treat Your Skin

I use a prescription retinoid cream to stop breakouts; I have since I was nineteen and had problematic skin. A side effect is that it's great for preventing fine lines. In a nutshell, it works by exfoliating your skin through renewing your surface cells at a much greater rate than they would ordinarily. This not only stops old and dead cells from accumulating on the surface and blocking your oil glands, but also keeps those fine lines from forming, which over time would turn into deeper lines. The prescription strength, which you'd need to get from a dermatologist, is much stronger than any over-the-counter retinol products you can buy, so start out with a low level, as retinoids can be drying at first.

If you use one, especially at prescription strength, you *must* wear sunscreen, because this kind of product makes your skin more susceptible to burns. (Of course, be sure to consult with your doctor if you're unsure!) Even though I'm now forty-six, to this day if I skip my retinoid cream two nights in a row, my skin starts to break out.

Even using this cream, I still have a spot or two on occasion that need extra help to avoid turning into a big pimple. Sometimes they do anyway. The best advice I have? Don't pick your zits. These days, if something turns into a bigger problem on my skin, it's almost always because I thought I could pop it—and I should know better by now!

If I see there might be tiny breakouts lurking that I can nip in the bud, I dab them with tamanu oil overnight. This oil has hydrating and anti-inflammatory properties, so it doesn't dry out your skin like an acne medication; it makes a zit go away without drying the skin around it. You can use it on any superficial redness or skin irritations too. It's pretty miraculous and like no other product I've ever used. On a recent Christmas movie shoot, I discovered that tamanu oil also works at staving off redness/dryness when you have a minor cold or allergies and have to blow your nose constantly. This is the absolute first time I can remember not having developed peeling, red, and irritated skin when having to blow my nose many times a day, and then having to follow each blow with copious foundation and powder touch-ups, all of which is super-hard on your skin. Tamanu oil truly is a miracle worker!

As for devices, I've seen results from one called the Perfectio Plus, which is rumored to count *Wonder Woman* Gal Gadot among its devotees. It's very costly but I have seen absolute results from it. (One of my best friends, Jen, got a two-for-one deal, and we each splurged on one.) It also comes with a lifetime guarantee. My only problem is remembering to use it! When I do, I notice the difference. The Perfectio uses infrared light to stimulate your skin in a similar way to a laser. For me, it's less effective for firming skin that's losing elasticity (a concern in my neck area) but absolutely reduces lines and appears to boost collagen production with consistent use.

Serums are also very helpful. Acetyl hexapeptide-3 (otherwise known as Argireline), Matrixyl 3000, and hyaluronic acid are clinically derived ingredients that help some people get results more similar to injections, smoothing the skin topically while allowing you to retain your full range of expressions. I love Arcona Peptide Hydrating Complex, and SkinRN Ultimate Hydration Serum (made in Nashville by my facialist here).

I think the key with any of these products is to mix it up, for skincare as well as food and supplements. And practitioners have told me this is true. Find several products you love that work well for you, and use them either in rotation (switch them every month, perhaps) or as you sense your skin (or body) needs.

Hydrate Your Skin

I love Arcona Magic Dry Ice and Epicuren Hydro Plus Moisture. I also love iS Clinical Copper Spray as a finisher for my skincare routine, as well as to lightly hold in place any makeup application, sprayed on top of it. It's a great refresher throughout the day as well. Another excellent skincare line is REN. Their products smell great and are very effective. I also love pure oil-based serums for added moisture; True Botanicals and Vintner's Daughter make some really great ones.

Protect Your Skin

I always wear a wide-brimmed hat when I'm gardening, but I don't stay *totally* out of the sun as I need vitamin D and it makes me feel good. But I protect myself because the most important external thing I can do for my skin is to use sunscreen religiously.

It's important to avoid chemical sunscreens, as their active ingredients (oxybenzone, octinoxate, and homosalate) can be endocrine disruptors and may cause cancer;[1] oxybenzone also kills coral reefs and is banned in Hawaii and other tropical places.[2] The active ingredients in mineral sunscreens are zinc oxide and titanium oxide, which are inert, nontoxic, and stay on the surface of your skin rather than being absorbed into your bloodstream as sunscreen chemicals are.[3]

I love iS Clinical Eclipse SPF 50 sunblock. It's mineral-based and very hydrating—it's effective sun protection with ingredients that are good for your skin. I put it on first thing every morning, whether I'll be outside in the sun or not. And it's a must-have for touchups if I'm filming outside—it was designed by a makeup artist, so it works beautifully both under or over foundation. As with any sunscreen, it should be reapplied every two to three hours, at minimum. Since I discovered it fourteen years ago, I haven't used anything else. It's the only sunscreen I've ever used that doesn't block my skin and protects me from sunburn.

Some of My Favorite Other Products

Hand cream: I love Jurlique Rose Hand Cream. It's the only rose-scented one I've tried that doesn't start smelling tinny or cloying after a bit, and it's also deeply moisturizing. If I put it on when I go to bed, my hands still smell good when I wake up. And so does Ernest after I rest my hand on him.

Lip balm: Ladybug Jane, which is vegan, organic, and super hydrating. It also tastes incredible and comes in flavors like sugar cookie, chocolate, mango, mint, and vanilla, among many others. Plus, it is about the most reasonably priced thing you could buy. It doesn't say so specifically, but it contains natural SPF as well.

Lip plumps: Add cinnamon powder or a few drops of cinnamon oil to your existing lip balm and plump your lips up yourself! You can also make a salt or sugar scrub using cinnamon mixed with some oil or melted cocoa butter.

Toothpaste: Nature's Gate Crème de Anise fluoride-free toothpaste or Hello toothpaste (in various fluoride-free configurations). I love the flavors, and since I've been using them, I haven't had any cavities (knock on wood!), and my hygienist and dentist tell me my teeth are in fantastic shape. I'd been nervous to use a non-fluoride product before, but so far it's working for me. I also like charcoal-based toothpastes, but you must utilize extreme caution when using them, or you'll end up with black splash-flecks everywhere! These products feel very good for my teeth and gums though, and definitely help to whiten if you brush for long enough.

Instant firming: I'm a big fan of the Spencer Barnes Neck and Face Wands. Spencer, who is a makeup artist in LA, designed these, and I can tell you they're truly effective. They're great for when you want instant results. They work best without anything under them, but you can also use the wands on top once your other products have been absorbed. These are great for days when I feel I need a boost, when I'm filming scenes I want to look extra refreshed for, or when doing press.

Facial masks: May Lindstrom's The Problem Solver is my go-to for a facial mask. It comes in a powder form, so you can mix it yourself—add a small amount of water and it's ready.

Body: A good everyday moisturizer for me is Jurlique Rose Body Lotion. I also really like cocoa butter as an occasional deep moisturizer. You can buy it by the bag, in solid chunks, and liquify it in a microwave or over some boiling water. For cleansing, I love the Nubian Heritage all-natural soaps. Their hemp & vetiver, coconut & papaya, and mango butter soaps all smell so good you want to eat them, and they do a great job of cleansing without irritating the skin or stripping natural oils.

Deodorant: I use Weleda Wild Rose 24H Deodorant Spray. I will tell you though, once in a while I go through a few days when it doesn't work! Without question, however, it has been the most effective and consistent natural deodorant I've ever used, though, and I'd much rather have an occasional day when it isn't working than put chemicals or aluminum on my sweat glands, near to so much that is tender and lymph nodes that are necessary to keep your immune system running the way it should. Fortunately, natural deodorant isn't very expensive, and if this brand doesn't work for you, try another.

Deodorants only prevent odor caused by the stinky bacteria in sweat. Unlike antiperspirants, they don't prevent sweating (which is a good thing—you're sweating because your body is cleansing itself). One reason natural deodorant may fail is if you wait too long after your shower to apply it. It's important that you wash your underarms last in the shower, dry off, and then apply your deodorant right away. And while you're figuring out which one is right for you, carry a tiny bit of perfumed oil with you, just in case it doesn't work!

Perfume: Lately, my day-to-day fragrance has simply been essential oils. Two that especially resonate for me are vetiver and geranium rose. I have two geranium rose plants in my house, and I've made my own oil from it—that's a lot of fun to experiment with! Rose geranium is a powerful energy cleanser, both in plant and in oil form.

Scent is so evocative. At times I've decided my character would have a specific fragrance, and I'll make an essential oil perfume for her. And then I feel totally different when I'm wearing it.

Throughout my life, since I first started having crushes, I've found vetiver to be my catnip when a potential love interest wears it. It makes me swoon—if I smell it, I start looking around to see who's wearing it because I instantly feel as though I want to make out with them! A few years ago, it finally dawned on me: If I love the fragrance so much and it's sexy to me, why don't I wear it myself? So now I mix a few drops of pure vetiver essential oil with some other oils and dab it on my pulse points. It always makes me feel both grounded and sensual.

Nail polish: I only use nail polish that is at least labelled "5-free," such as

Zoya. But now you can find polish that's 8- or even 10-free, and it lasts just as long, with a lot less toxic scent when you're applying it.

Insect repellent: I'm a magnet for mosquitos, but I've found that lemon eucalyptus oil, if slathered on thick, keeps them off me. (I do use commercial sprays when going into a thickly infested area, but I try to avoid DEET, and always shower it off before going to bed.)

Candles: I love candles, but I try to stick to sustainably sourced, plant-based ones, fragranced only with natural oils. Look for "pthalate-free" and "100%" in the wax description, or you know they're using a combination of other ingredients they don't want to tell you about. Since the candle burns directly into the air you breathe, being mindful of what they're made of seems really important to me. The jury is still out as to whether paraffin wax leaves more soot in your air or not, but I figure, why take a chance when you can easily (and affordably) avoid it?

My Hair Routine

Up to the time I starred in *Fun*, my dad had been the only one to trim my hair. So when I learned I was going to the Sundance Festival, I went to Supercuts because I had no idea where else to go, and asked them give me a cleanup on the ends of my very long hair. No layering, no styling. That was a big deal for me. My hair had been so long my entire life, and I was going to an actual salon! After that, for several years I didn't do anything with my hair; it remained straight and long (and always red—I've still never colored it!).

During the second season of *Cybill*, an industry hair pro gave me a great cut, and this was the beginning of my learning I could have different hairstyles—and how layers can give your hair movement and make it look a lot thicker. When I cut it short for the first time, right after I filmed *Two Weeks Notice*, my mom cried when she saw me. But by the end of that visit, she said, "I have to admit your hair's pretty cute!"

Don't Overdo It with Styling and Products

My hair-care routine is incredibly simple: I don't style my hair when I'm not working. I have to admit, I'm terrible at it. I don't know how to use a round brush and am not planning to learn, and I have no intention of spending a lot of time with styling products when there's so much else I'd rather do!

On the set, my hair often gets a lot done to it, which can be drying and damaging, and the heat of the bright lights makes things worse. Unless I'm playing a character who's severely uptight and it's part of the look, I'm constantly asking the hair department to make things looser. I prefer that my hair doesn't look *too* styled.

So I try to leave my hair alone as much as possible in between shoots. I shower at least once a day (unless we're in a pandemic lockdown, and then all bets are off!), but I don't need to wash my hair every day; it's not good for it anyway. If it isn't dirty, I pull it back in a ponytail and put a hairband over the front of it, so it doesn't get wet in the shower. When I do wash it, I'm a big fan of letting my hair air-dry.

Usually, I use the reasonably priced thickening shampoo and conditioner by Davines, which a hairstylist on one of my Hallmark movies told me about. I have a lot of hair, but it's fine, so volumizing products are helpful. No matter what, I always try to shampoo with sulfate-free products. For extra conditioning, if my hair has been styled on set every day, once a week I apply a lot of coconut oil and let it soak in while I sleep. As long as I don't do this more often, I find it effective, and my hair is much softer when I (thoroughly!) wash it out. You can also buy inexpensive and effective packs of specially formulated oils at the drugstore. Apply to your hair and top with a shower cap while sleeping, and you'll wake up with magically well-conditioned hair.

For styling, an easy 'do is to use a bit of Bumble and Bumble Surf Spray throughout. The ocean-y texture makes your hair look like you've spent a day in the waves. Especially when my hair is shorter, I work a styling cream into the ends and a tad more through the rest of my hair; applying when my hair has air-dried a bit. I flip upside down to encourage my hair to curl and develop some body, and it does something vaguely presentable on its own at that point. (She said hopefully...) A light shine spray once it dries can help if it looks lifeless. If I have to blow-dry my hair, I use mousse at the base to add volume and protection. Kevin Murphy, Rusk, and Davines styling products are some of my favorite brands.

Dry shampoo has been a game changer. I love the powder shake-on ones from Aveda (Shampure), which gives me a lift at the roots and base and absorbs excess oils there, and the sprays from Drybar and Rusk, which are especially good for oily places like bangs or wisps of hair framing your face. (Be mindful not to breathe in the dry shampoo. I spray it while holding my breath, and then walk away from the cloud.) As I mentioned, I prefer not to wash my hair every day if I can help it, so dry shampoo can often save a hairstyle from one day to another, not only cutting down on the wear and tear on your hair but also saving you time. I typically don't pin it all up into neat curls even if I'm trying to save it. Most nights, I gather my hair in a ponytail holder and kind of bunch it at my crown so it's not under my neck as I sleep. Sometimes I fall asleep with wet hair (not a good idea if it's cold where you're sleeping, but a good idea otherwise!) and wake up with natural ringlets.

People often tell me my hair looks pretty and that they wished their own hair looked like mine. That always surprises me because I don't do much of anything to it most of the time! To be sure, I've always said I'm lucky to be a redhead, because it masks the actual hot mess that my hair often is. However, I do think the fact that I don't style it with heat and heavy combing/brushing when I'm not working helps it stay healthier. If you're someone who routinely styles your hair a specific way, I bet you've had the experience where one day you run out of time, letting it go naturally, and then everyone tells you how gorgeous your natural hair is. (I'm thinking of my girlfriends and how stunning their hair looks when it's minimally styled or air-dried out of the shower.) It's so much fun to go to a salon and get a blowout or play around with styling your hair, but I'm an advocate for doing less. And of course, a low-maintenance approach will save you time!

Try No-Suds Shampoo

Since *The Walking Dead* is set during a zombie apocalypse, hair styling (ideally) shouldn't be evident. It's the only show I've ever done where hair and makeup takes all of thirty minutes total, if that! I had to make my fine hair not look like it was frizzed out from washing it all the time, but also not oily, and also not styled. Karen, the key hairstylist, had the perfect solution: DevaCurl No-Poo Original Zero Lather Conditioning Cleanser. As the name implies, it doesn't suds up; it's kind of a nourishing lotion, and you don't need conditioner with it. You massage it in, let it sit while you wash the rest of your body, rinse it out, and presto: clean hair without the "squeaky clean" that normally means it's been stripped with harsher cleanser. I don't know exactly how it works, but it somehow does. Plus, it helps bring down any frizz, so you don't need as many styling products. I've had No-Poo on my shower shelf ever since, and I use it at least once a week in lieu of shampoo. And something about it still reminds me of washing my hair with it in the tiny motel shower in Peachtree City, where I stayed while working on that show; getting up first thing in the morning to prepare for the ride in to set; and the singularly thrilling, satisfying, life-changing experience I had during my short time there.

PART V

The

recipes

CHAPTER 9

Small Changes Recipes

Just another city sidewalk
summer night making small talk
Cobblestones and conversation
thank you for the wine

—"DOWN SHE GOES"

haven't always been an expert at cooking, lest you get the wrong idea. And I hardly consider myself an expert now—I'm merely someone who has collected a lot of experience and has a whole lot of fun making delicious food for myself and others!

When my first boyfriend, Peter, and I had just moved in together, we invited my dear friend Robert over for dinner to celebrate the new house we were renting. It was owned by Sharon Stone and had been her home when *Basic Instinct*, her big break, came out. Because her trajectory from working actor in the 1980s to well-recognized actor in *Total Recall* to overnight superstar happened so suddenly, she had to contend with some obsessive fans. Since she'd owned her home long before this was a problem, her address was public record. After a number of unwanted visitors, she was so afraid for her security that she installed corrugated steel shutters which, at the touch of a switch, concealed every door and window in the house. And there were *lots* of floor-to-ceiling windows in the back, overlooking the most surreally gorgeous view of the San Fernando Valley. I'll never forget the feeling of closing all the electronic shutters at night, as though simply because the shutters were there, the house needed to be transformed into a windowless box before going to bed. It certainly felt safe though!

So when we had Robert over to celebrate our cohabitation in Sharon Stone's steel fortress, I decided I'd try my hand at making garlic mashed potatoes, one of my favorite things. I should add that Robert and I both absolutely loved garlic; many things bonded us, but our mutual ravenous love for garlic was a cementing factor of our friendship. When The Stinking Rose opened in LA, we were there the very first night. They brought us table bread in a basket, with whole roasted garlic cloves doused in so much oil they were the consistency of drawn butter, to spread on our slices. We finished the whole basket and asked for more. Whatever our main course was, it was slathered in garlic—knowing my diet at the time, my protein was likely roast chicken—with garlic mashed potatoes and garlic spinach on the side. The topper was dessert—vanilla ice cream with chocolate mole sauce—and garlic infused both the ice cream and the chocolate. We'd never been made happier by a meal, and we left the restaurant full of garlic (and yes, flatulence—I remember us gleefully talking on the phone about how farty we were).

Early the next morning at my orthodontist's appointment, I waited for a moment in the exam chair with my back to the door. When my orthodontist walked in, before I even saw his face, he said, "Garlic last night?" I was mortified! He could smell it all the way from the door. Before he would adjust my braces, he found some BreathAsure and had me take them, letting them digest first. (The embarrassment was totally worth it. Twenty-five years on, I can still taste that dinner.)

I wanted to create some garlic mashed potatoes that would be reminiscent of that incredible meal at The Stinking Rose. What I didn't yet realize is that garlic must be *cooked* before being added to potatoes. Duh! Well, Robert took a bite and he asked, tentatively, "Did you cook this garlic?"

"Was I supposed to?" I replied.

Robert tried not to laugh, and he and Peter both ate a few more bites to be polite. And to this day, Robert *still* brings up my Raw Garlic Mashed Potatoes!

(*Note:* When I make mashed potatoes now, I either use garlic powder to make them garlicky, or I add wasabi paste. I might like wasabi mash even better!)

Have Fun with Substitutions

With these recipes you'll see that the only difference between them and non-vegan meals is that dairy, meat, poultry, fish, and eggs aren't used—and if you're anything like the non-vegan eaters I love to prepare food for, you won't miss them because you'll be too busy enjoying how delicious everything tastes!

It's incredibly easy to alter your favorite recipes and make them vegan—or otherwise modify them for whatever goals you may have, vegan or not—with only a few adjustments. You may need to adjust cooking times, depending on the water content of the ingredients you're substituting or the oil profile. But those are simple tweaks.

Here are a few basic substitutions for your primary ingredients:

For meat, poultry, or fish: Use vegan "meat," tempeh, seitan, extra-firm tofu, mushrooms (portabello, cremini, shiitake, or oyster), or beans, depending on the consistency of the ingredient called for.

For dairy: Use vegan dairy substitutes, such as oat milk, rice milk, or a plethora of nut milk options, sweetened or unsweetened; tofu; or coconut yogurts (like Siggi's, which is only lightly sweetened). I use Daiya or Violife plant-based "cheese." (Quality plant-based cheeses truly melt these days, and many are just protein and oil, not necessarily soy or nut-laden.) Instead of butter, use Earth Balance or Miyoko's plant-based butter. Coconut oil or a good extra-virgin olive oil often serves as a great substitute too.

For eggs: Use Just Egg plant-based scramble, applesauce, tofu, white beans, mashed chickpeas, or even the liquid from a can of chickpeas (called aquafaba), depending on what kind of egg you need in the recipe. In baking, an egg substitute can be as simple as whisking together a ratio of one tablespoon of water to one teaspoon of ground flaxseed and letting the mixture, usually called a "flax egg," sit for a few seconds.

"Traditional" Lasagna, Meat and Dairy Free

When I moved into my first solo apartment, as a housewarming gift, my dad sent me *The Betty Crocker Cookbook*. I was just figuring out how to cook things I hadn't made before, and this book teaches the basics—even how to boil water! I often made its lasagna, as lasagna had been one of my favorite dinners since I was little (and still is). Given the strict diet I grew up on, my dad's version of it had been delicious, but as my diet expanded, it was definitely on the blander side—no salt, no spices. So I was excited to have a tried-and-true recipe to turn to.

At first, I swapped out the ground meat/pork for ground turkey, since I didn't eat red meat by that point. Next, after I'd decided to remove poultry from my diet, I subbed the meat/pork with Smart Ground vegan meat substitute, back when that was the only real ground meat substitute on the market. Then, I substituted plant-based options for the cheese and egg, and started using gluten-free rice noodles for my friends who are gluten-free. And now, you can even find green lentil lasagna noodles. (Or, if you have time on your hands, you could make homemade lasagna noodles. These are one of the easiest noodles to hand make because they require just a rolling pin and a knife. No fancy shapes!)

Regular Lasagna	Plant-Based Lasagna
Ground beef, pork, and/ or Italian sausage	"Meat," like Beyond Burger
Parmesan	Dairy-free parmesan
Mozzarella	Daiya or Violife mozzarella
Ricotta	Tofu or cashew ricotta (homemade)

Tip #1: I also like to add mushrooms, sautéed with a bit of dry red wine and anise seeds, to the "meat" mix. You'll see Paula's Bolognegeze (not a typo!) recipe later in this chapter; if you really want to make a special meat sauce, you can use that in any lasagna.

Tip #2: To make cashew ricotta, soak two cups of cashews in water and cover for eight hours to soften them. Drain. Blend to make them smooth, but not until they turn to cashew butter. Add a bit of water, a couple of tablespoons of lemon juice, nutritional yeast, dill, parsley, salt and pepper—voilà! You can also make tofu ricotta by using the same approximate amount of extra-firm tofu, drained and crumbled. You'll find specific instructions for making a nice combo of the two under my zucchini lasagna recipe on page 235, but the fun thing about both of these is that you almost can't go wrong. If your "ricotta" is too bland, you can easily season it. Start with less water, since you can always add more if your ricotta is too crumbly, but you can't as easily take it out.

I also recommend preparing more soaked cashews than you think you'll need. If you end up with too few, you won't have time to soak cashews for eight hours when you're in the middle of assembling your lasagna. If you end up with too many, you can save the extras or use them to make cashew cream or cashew milk. Cream is made by putting the soaked cashews in your blender and adding water until it just covers the tops of them; you can use this as a creamer for soups, as a coffee creamer, or in various desserts. Or, for a simple nut milk, place the cashews in a blender, add water to cover about two inches above them, and blend until liquified.

Greens in a Pinch

You can even make substitutions/enhancements to a recipe you already know and love, to suit your existing food lifestyle. Here's an example from my own life:

Nashville had a massive windstorm six weeks after the 2019 tornado, and the electricity unexpectedly went out for twenty-four hours at the rental I was living in while my house was being repaired. I'd emptied the fridge and freezer by then, so I had no fresh groceries in the house, and it was storming so hard I didn't even want to try for a take-out delivery. But I wanted greens anyway. I made a super-easy adaptation of Daiya's boxed mac and cheese, which I had in the pantry.

- As the pasta was cooking per the instructions on the box (I always go a minute less for al dente pasta), I prepared the sauce.
- In a bowl, I mixed one tablespoon spirulina powder and one scoop (included in the container) of Amazing Grass Supergreens. I then took a few scoops of boiling, salted water from the pasta pot and used a fork to whisk it with the powders until smooth.
- Next, I added the cheese sauce and whisked again until smooth. (Pretty too!)
- When the pasta was done, I drained it and added it to the sauce. It made enough for two servings.

So delicious and full of green nutrients. I'm eating my leftovers as I type, and I can confirm that they're absolutely delicious cold.

Breakfast

Avocado Toast

Here is a spin I've never seen before on this popular breakfast item. I discovered it by accident, and I love the way the kiwi makes the avocado spread even greener.

> 1 small avocado, peeled, pitted, and sliced
> ½ kiwi, peeled and sliced
> Pinch of Himalayan sea salt
> Sprinkle of ground tarragon
> 2 slices Ezekiel bread

Mash all the ingredients together and serve on toast.
Yields 2 slices of avo toast

Perfect Green Smoothie

I make some sort of version of this most days, varying wildly in ingredients based on what I've got sitting around. Now, I don't mind a really hearty smoothie filled with whatever healthy produce I have on hand (that's code for *I wouldn't serve this to anyone but myself*) but when I made this one, I did a little happy dance and immediately wrote down exactly what I did. Because it was perfect!

> 12 ounces Harmless Harvest coconut water
>
> A handful each of fresh parsley and cilantro
>
> 2 handfuls fresh spinach leaves
>
> 1 "finger" fresh turmeric root
>
> 1/2 teaspoon spirulina powder
>
> 1/2 banana, previously frozen
>
> 1/3 cup frozen mango chunks
>
> 1 scoop vanilla protein powder (my favorite is Four Sigmatic; Orgain and PlantFusion also work well)
>
> 1 scoop Amazing Grass Green Superfood
>
> 1/2 teaspoon each Host Defense Reishi and Turkey Tail mushroom powders, optional (or substitute any mushroom-based immunity-boosting powder)
>
> 3 dates, pits removed

Place all the ingredients in a blender and use the liquify setting until the smoothie is free of any lumps.

Yields approximately 3 cups (enough for a satisfying meal, or split in half for two, and serve with a light snack)

Scrambled Beans

I started making scrambled beans for myself quite a while ago. I don't remember how I came up with the idea, but once I did, it was kind of a no-brainer. Why wouldn't you make scrambled beans? Even though I enjoy eggs on occasion, I much prefer my beans, as they're a great source of iron and fiber. And I love how they taste!

Also, if you're eating out, many restaurants don't think to have beans on their breakfast menu, but they're likely to have them in the kitchen, so they can make them for you. Ask for a side of avocado and some sautéed greens, or a piece of toast or side of fruit to go with them, and you're good to go.

> 2 teaspoons coconut oil
> 1 carton cannellini beans
> ¼ cup water, plus extra
> ¼ cup nutritional yeast
> 1 teaspoon garlic powder
> ½ teaspoon onion powder
> ½ teaspoon turmeric powder
> Dash of paprika
> ¼ cup vegan cheddar shreds
> Pinch of salt

Combine the coconut oil and beans in a medium skillet over low heat and stir until the oil is blended with the beans. Add about ¼ cup of water. Bring to a simmer, then add the nutritional yeast. While cooking, add the turmeric, paprika, onion powder, and garlic powder. Add a bit more water as the beans start to become more dry; don't allow all the water to evaporate until the beans have cooked and become creamy, for about seven minutes. When done, turn the heat off, immediately add the "cheddar," and stir until melted. Grind a little salt over it to taste, stir, and serve.

Note: You can also make a wrap out of these using collard greens. Place the leaf shiny-side down on the plate, then put your fillings in the center. Fold the top and bottom in first, then roll the left and right sides. Flip the wrap upside down; let the heat soften the leaf a bit before eating, which will make it less likely to fall apart.

The leaf will also hold better and be more flexible if it has been allowed to wilt ever so slightly first. If I'm not using collards right away, I like to store them in a cup of water in the refrigerator, with the stems intact. But you'll want to take them out of the water, or pick them, at least fifteen minutes before you wrap with them or they'll be very crunchy—still super delicious but messier (she said knowingly).

Yields 2 servings

Superfood Pancakes

I love sneaking healthy ingredients into things that, on the surface, look like they're a treat rather than health food. *Why can't a pancake be both a treat and healthy?* I wondered. So I set to work inventing. This pancake also reminds me of buttermilk pancakes, which used to be a favorite of mine. The idea to combine banana and rosemary came by accident. I had some overripe bananas in my fruit bowl on the counter next to some sprigs of fresh rosemary I'd just picked. A waft of both scents met me while I was cleaning up after cooking dinner, and I instantly got excited to taste those flavors together.

$1/8$ cup quinoa flour

$1/8$ cup coconut flour

$1/8$ cup unflavored pure pea protein (like Whole Foods' 365 brand)

$1/4$ cup Bob's Red Mill Gluten Free 1-to-1 Baking Flour

$1 1/2$ teaspoons baking powder

$1/4$ teaspoon maca powder

$1/8$ teaspoon ground cardamom

$1/4$ teaspoon Himalayan sea salt

$1/2$ cup almond milk

2 1/2 tablespoons water

2 1/4 teaspoons aquafaba (page 201)

1 1/2 teaspoons vanilla

1 heaping tablespoon maple syrup (plus more for serving)

1 teaspoon lemon juice

1 1/2 tablespoons coconut oil, liquified (plus more for griddle)

1 very ripe banana, thinly sliced

Approximately 40 fresh rosemary leaves (minced if preferred—
taste is the same!)

Miyoko's "butter" for garnish (if desired)

Combine the quinoa flour, coconut flour, pea protein, baking flour, baking powder, maca powder, cardamom, and sea salt in an electric mixer (preferable) or whisk by hand. In a separate bowl, combine the almond milk, water, aquafaba, vanilla, maple syrup, lemon juice, and coconut oil, being sure to add liquified coconut oil last (you can microwave it for 15 to 20 seconds if it's too firm). Mix together with a small electric hand mixer or whisk by hand. With the large mixer running, add the liquid to the dry and mix on low, working up to high, till the mix is sticky and pancake-batter-like.

Heat a GreenPan griddle on medium-low for at least 3 minutes, with coconut oil rubbed over the surface with a paper towel. When the oil is lightly hot (separating into little pools on the surface), put the pancake batter in, 2 pancakes at a time, in 1/4 cup scoops. Then add about 5 banana slices and sprinkle 8 to 10 loose leaves of rosemary per pancake.

When the edges start lifting up, about 4 to 5 minutes, carefully flip the pancakes over. (Cooking times may vary based on your stovetop and your pan; if the pancake isn't yet ready to flip, let it be a bit longer!) Cook for another 2 minutes and then put on a plate, flipping again to serve, banana side up. Serve with maple syrup and a pat of Miyoko's plant-based butter, if desired.

Note: I also tried making this recipe with Four Sigmatic's excellent superfoods protein powder, which is packed with adaptogenic and immune-boosting mushrooms, as well as multiple sources of plant protein. I definitely prefer the consistency of the pea protein pancakes. However, the superfoods protein gave the pancakes an also-delicious whole-grain or buckwheat sort of vibe. I'd recommend trying both!
Yields 4 pancakes, or 2 servings

Thank-You-God Granola

I've been making granola for a long time, off and on, but in the past I always made it with honey, which helps it stick to itself. I'm a (mostly) plant-based eater who doesn't have a problem with ethically sourced honey, but some vegans don't use it. Also, I didn't want to use nut butter, since some people have nut allergies. My challenge was not in getting it to taste good, but in making it have those sought-after clusters. After no fewer than eight tries—the absolute most of any recipe in this book!—I literally prayed for this to turn out. And it did! No kidding, I couldn't even sleep at night while I was trying to get this one right. I hope you enjoy it. It's not too sweet, not too spicy, and not too crunchy—but it crunches and, yes siree Bob, it has clusters. Hallelujah!

  1 tablespoon ground flax meal
  3 tablespoons water
  3 tablespoons coconut oil
  3 tablespoons maple syrup
  1 tablespoon vanilla
  1 1/2 cup oats

¾ cup coconut flakes

2 tablespoons coconut flour

¼ cup coconut sugar

2 tablespoons hemp seeds

1 teaspoon ground cinnamon

¾ teaspoon Himalayan sea salt

½ teaspoon ground nutmeg

¼ teaspoon ground ginger

2 tablespoons pecans (or substitute pumpkin seeds if you have
   a nut allergy)

3 tablespoons dried blueberries

3 chopped dried figs

Preheat the oven to 300 degrees.

Make the flax "egg" by beating the flax meal and water together in a separate small bowl, using a fork or small hand mixer. Set aside.

In a separate small bowl, mix the coconut oil, maple syrup, and vanilla. Microwave for 15 seconds if necessary to soften the coconut oil, although you don't need to liquify it.

In a large bowl, mix together the oats, coconut flakes, coconut flour, coconut sugar, hemp seeds, cinnamon, Himalayan sea salt, nutmeg, and ginger. Add the coconut oil/maple syrup mix and blend thoroughly, coating all the dry ingredients. Add the pecans/pumpkin seeds and blueberries/figs and mix again to combine. Finally, add the flax mixture, mixing again with your hands, if possible, to be sure that it evenly coats everything.

Put a sheet of parchment paper on a cookie sheet. Put the granola on it in an even layer, though not so thin that you can see the sheet through the oats. (You want it to stick to itself slightly.) Bake for 15 minutes, take out and check to be sure it's not getting too brown in places, as oven temps vary. Put the cookie sheet back in for 20 minutes, checking the granola every 10 minutes. If it does start to get too brown, turn those places, but the less you stir it, the more it will form into those sought-after clusters! Remove from the oven and allow the granola to cool completely before breaking it apart and storing it in a mason jar or glass container. Will keep fresh in the cupboard unrefrigerated for a month at least, and it can be stored in the fridge longer.

Note: If crunchiness is more important to you than clusters, go ahead and stir at the 15-minute mark, and you can cook it for an extra 5–10 minutes as long as it's not burning!

Yields approximately 4 cups of granola

Tofu Scramble with Sautéed Spinach and Ezekiel Bread ∞∞∞∞∞∞∞∞

You can serve this with sliced fruit and half an avocado, if you like. You also can substitute one teaspoon of turmeric powder for the curry powder and fresh turmeric. I happened to make the recipe this way because of ingredients I did and didn't have—and I loved how it turned out.

8 ounces extra-firm tofu, drained

2 tablespoons nutritional yeast

1/2 teaspoon ground cumin

1/2 teaspoon dried dill

1/2 teaspoon tarragon powder

1 tablespoon finely minced fresh turmeric root, peeled
   (or 1 teaspoon dried powder)

Dash of red pepper flakes

Dash of curry powder, optional (to pump up the color)

1 teaspoon coconut oil

¼ onion, chopped

Himalayan sea salt, to taste

3 cremini, shiitake, or white button mushrooms, sliced

2 garlic cloves, sliced

2 cups spinach

1 teaspoon olive oil

Dash of garlic powder

¼ cup vegan mozzarella

Freshly ground black pepper

1 teaspoon chopped cilantro

1 teaspoon chopped chives

2 slices Ezekiel bread

2 scrapes of vegan butter and/or preserves of your choice

In a medium bowl, crumble together the tofu, nutritional yeast, cumin, dill, tarragon, turmeric root, red pepper flakes, and curry powder. In a GreenPan, sauté the onion on low-medium heat with 1 teaspoon coconut oil (don't heat the oil first). Add a grind or two of salt and cook until the onions are translucent. Add the mushrooms and garlic and cook until fragrant. Add the tofu mixture and cook for 10 minutes on low/medium heat. Put the Ezekiel bread in a toaster and set to medium. In a separate skillet, sauté the spinach with the olive oil and a dash each of salt and garlic powder. Cook on low/medium until the spinach is wilted, then add the vegan mozzarella to the scramble. Season with freshly ground black pepper and another dash of salt, if needed. Sprinkle cilantro and chives over the scramble. Spread a scrape of vegan butter and/or preserves over each slice of Ezekiel bread. Plate the tofu and the spinach, and serve with a slice of bread.

Yields 2 servings

Lunch and Dinner

Soups

Cream of Broccoli Soup

As you know by now, broccoli is one of my favorite things, and so is cream. I've tried many different vegan recipes for this, namely from *The Conscious Cook* and *Oh She Glows* cookbooks, as well as non-vegan ones back when I still ate dairy, and over the years, here's how I have learned to throw it together without overthinking it. It's a wonderfully easy but fancy-looking and tasting thing to get going on the stove when someone is dropping by for dinner unexpectedly.

    ½ teaspoon Himalayan sea salt (plus more for pan)
    ½ medium onion, chopped
    1 tablespoon coconut oil
    1 clove garlic, chopped
    1 stalk celery, chopped
    1 very large broccoli crown (approximately 2 cups when
        chopped)
    Cracked black pepper to taste (8 grinds, approximately
        ¼ teaspoon)
    Juice from ½ a lemon
    1 ½ tablespoons parsley, chopped
    1 ½ tablespoons oregano, chopped
    3 cups low-sodium vegetable broth
    1 cup cashew cream (page 202)
    25 fresh basil leaves
    Handful raw spinach leaves

1 tablespoon nutritional yeast

Vegan cheddar cheese shreds (for topping)

In a large saucepan, add 4 grinds of Himalayan sea salt and heat on medium for 30 seconds. Add the onion and coconut oil, cook for 2 minutes, then add the garlic. Cook for another 5 minutes on medium or until onion is translucent. Add the celery and broccoli; cover and cook on medium-low for another 5 minutes. Add Himalayan sea salt, pepper, lemon juice, parsley, and oregano; cook another 3 minutes. Add the low-sodium vegetable broth, increase the heat to medium, and cover and cook for another 20 minutes, keeping an eye on the liquid level.

Add the cashew cream, then cook another 5 minutes on medium-low.

Transfer the soup to a blender. Add the basil, spinach, and nutritional yeast. With a hand towel covering the blender lid (to avoid hot splashes), blend starting on low, then slowly increase to the highest speed, until the soup is completely liquified.

Serve topped with a sprinkle of vegan cheddar cheese shreds.

Yields 2 large bowls, or 4 appetizer bowls

Cream of Tomato Soup

I remember how much I loved the comfort of cream of tomato soup when I did eat dairy, so I wanted to create a dairy-free version. I honestly don't think anyone would be able to tell the difference.

1 tablespoon olive oil

1 medium onion, chopped coarsely

2 medium heirloom tomatoes (or other varieties), peeled

2 cloves garlic, chopped

2 stalks celery, coarsely chopped

20 cherry tomatoes, any variety, halved

8 grinds Himalayan sea salt

12 grinds black pepper

2 long stalks rosemary, sprigs only

1/8 teaspoon ground cardamom

1/2 cup coconut milk (full-fat)

Sauté the onion on medium heat in large saucepan until translucent. Peel the tomatoes by submerging them in a pot of boiling water for 2 minutes, then plunging them into a large bowl prefilled with ice and water. After they cool, roll off their skins, core, and chop coarsely. Add the tomatoes to the onions. Add the garlic, celery, cherry tomatoes, sea salt, black pepper, rosemary, and cardamom. Cook together for another 10 to 15 minutes, until everything turns a nice tomato-soup color. Add the coconut milk and stir all together, another minute or so. Put the mixture into a blender, with a hand towel covering the blender lid (to avoid hot splashes). Start on low speed and gradually increase to the highest speed.

Yields enough for 4 appetizer portions, or 2 larger bowls of soup

Gazpacho

This is an especially satisfying thing to make if you've grown your own tomatoes and cucumbers and you're wondering what to do with them all!

4 pounds heirloom tomatoes (approximately 8 medium), peeled

1 jumbo or 2 medium cucumbers, peeled and sliced
   (approximately 2 cups)

12 grinds Himalayan sea salt

14 grinds black pepper

Approximately ½ cup fresh cilantro (loose leaves)

1 cup fresh basil (loosely chopped)

¼ cup olive oil

Chopped avocado and tomato, for garnish

Peel the tomatoes by submerging them in a pot of boiling water for 2 minutes, then plunging them into a large bowl prefilled with ice and water. After they cool, roll off their skins, core, and chop coarsely. Put the tomatoes, cucumbers, sea salt, black pepper, cilantro, and basil into a blender, and blend until liquified. With the blender running, at a slightly reduced speed to minimize splashing, slowly add the olive oil (otherwise the oil will separate). Chill at least 3 hours. Shake or stir well before pouring the soup into bowls. Serve with chopped avocado and fresh tomato and the drizzle.

Yields 3 to 4 starter servings, or 2 larger ones

Drizzle

2 cherry tomatoes

1 tablespoon olive oil

2 grinds Himalayan sea salt

5 bunches fresh basil

Put the cherry tomatoes, olive oil, sea salt, and basil into a food processor and blend until liquified as much as possible. Strain the liquid out either with a fine mesh strainer or a cheesecloth, and use the strained liquid as garnish for the gazpacho.

Note: If you make this soup in a blender other than a Vitamix, you may end up with a chunkier gazpacho. It still tastes great! My preference here is for the silkiest, smoothest texture.

Sweet Potato Soup with Sage and Turmeric

Little did I know the first year I planted sweet potatoes in my Nashville garden that eighteen tiny sweet potato plants will grow five to seven sweet potatoes per plant, with each crop requiring digging up to two feet into the ground, chasing one to the next, like some sort of grossly mis-shapen Mardi Gras beads belonging in a giant's jewelry box. So the next year I cut back and only planted twelve in April. I didn't pull them up till November and ended up with sweet potatoes as big as my forearm (no exaggeration—see the photo in the insert). Many of them were delicious, and I had to quickly come up with lots of creative ways to use them. For-tunately, this soup keeps well in the freezer and can easily be heated up when you want to eat it.

1 tablespoon coconut oil

2 small yellow onions

2 cloves garlic

2 celery stalks, chopped

1 medium Fuji apple, peeled and chopped

2 tablespoons maple syrup

1 carton vegetable broth

1 can coconut milk (I prefer full-fat, but low-fat is fine if you want a lighter soup)

1 generous handful sage leaves, chopped

6 medium/large sweet potatoes, peeled and coarsely chopped

Nutmeg, chili powder, Himalayan sea salt, and ground black pepper to taste

1 large "finger" turmeric root, peeled and coarsely chopped (if you can't find fresh, use 1 tablespoon ground turmeric instead)

Juice of 1 lime

1 to 2 tablespoons chopped cilantro

Heat the coconut oil in a large saucepan for one minute on medium heat. Add the onion and sauté for three minutes. Add the garlic, celery, and apple and sauté for five minutes. Add the maple syrup, coat everything well, and sauté for another two minutes. Add the vegetable broth, coconut milk, sage leaves, and sweet potatoes. Season with the nutmeg, chili powder, Himalayan sea salt, and ground black pepper to taste (½ teaspoon of each is a good place to start). Cook for another fifteen minutes, until the potatoes are very soft. Transfer to a Vitamix or blender in batches, so the container is half-full each time. Add even amounts of the turmeric and lime juice to each batch before blending. Covering the lid with a hand towel (to avoid hot splashes), start on low, increasing speed to high to liquify.

Yields 2 to 4 servings

Salads

Chickpea Salad (Mock Tuna Salad)

This is equally delicious in a wrap, with a couple of slices of avocado, or atop a bed of greens. You can also turn this into a mock tuna melt by adding any bread of your choice and "cheese" slices, then cooking it like a grilled cheese sandwich.

1 (29-ounce) can or 2 (15-ounce) cans chickpeas, drained

8 grinds black pepper

2 tablespoons Vegenaise

Juice from 1 lemon

1 teaspoon tarragon powder

1 teaspoon onion powder

Dash chili powder

1 heaping tablespoon chives, chopped

1 heaping tablespoon parsley, minced

1 1/2 tablespoons nutritional yeast

1/2 teaspoon Himalayan sea salt

1/4 cup finely chopped celery, optional

Put all the chickpeas into a bowl, then add the pepper, Vegenaise, lemon juice, tarragon, onion powder, chili powder, chives, parsley, nutritional yeast, and sea salt, stirring each one to mix before adding the next. Using a potato masher or a large fork, mash the chickpeas and seasonings until about three-quarters of the chickpeas are mashed, leaving the others whole. Add the celery, if using, and serve. The salad will keep fresh for at least 3 days in the fridge.

Note: You can wrap this in a collard leaf wrap (or two) for a wonderfully balanced lunch. See note on collards on page 206.

Yields 4 generous scoop-size servings

Kale Salad

This is a salad where only kale will do. Rubbing avocado on some of the more delicate greens won't quite work the same, since they aren't as crunchy (and chopping them wouldn't be as effective either). However, if you love salad but kale isn't your favorite, please try this with spinach, collards, chard, beet greens, or arugula. You won't be able to mash the avocado in the same way, but you could still create a delicious "dressing" with the half avocado, salt, pepper, and a splash of water in a blender, and pour it over them. Variety is key. For some people, kale is harder to digest than these other greens.

1 1/2 cups kale, chopped

1/2 avocado, peeled, pitted, and sliced

1 beefsteak tomato, chopped

Himalayan sea salt and ground black pepper, to taste

Mix the greens and the avocado together, mashing as you go. Add the tomato, and salt and black pepper to taste.

Yields 1 serving

Warm Spinach and Beyond Burger Salad

This recipe is also something I threw together that I thought was especially tasty. It's an example of how easy it can be to make inventive, crave-worthy lunches when your fridge is stocked with delicious ingredients.

3 cups raw spinach leaves, torn by hand a bit
   (with clean hands!)

1/2 to 1 ripe mango, cut into 1 1/2-inch cubes

1/2 avocado, peeled, pitted, and sliced

Aged balsamic vinegar

1 teaspoon extra-virgin olive oil

1 Beyond Burger

1 cup roasted sweet potato slices

Himalayan sea salt and ground black pepper, to taste

Place the spinach in a large mixing bowl. Add the mango, avocado, a few dashes of the vinegar, and the extra-virgin olive oil. In a small frying pan, cook the Beyond Burger as directed. When you flip it, add the roasted sweet potato slices to the pan. Heat together for 3 minutes in the juices from the burger. Add a dash of olive oil if needed. When the burger is cooked, break it into chunks with a spatula, then add it and the sweet potatoes to the salad. Toss well, until the heat begins to wilt the spinach. Use 2 grinds of the salt and 3 grinds of the pepper. Serve immediately. *Yields 1 serving*

Wild Violets and Greens Salad

Wild violets, along with many other incredible medicinal "weeds," grow plentifully in Nashville, and throughout many places. I love the flavor and beauty of violets, and many other edible and medicinal wild weeds are out there—including the common dandelion, which is a powerful liver cleanser. Make sure you consult with an expert before you decide something is edible (mine is my friend Kim Collins, East Nashville healer and natural medicine guru, who makes incredible tinctures and body balms from wild medicinals she harvests in her backyard). Violets are pretty easy to spot, but several weeds have look-alikes that are toxic, so if you're in doubt, don't eat it!

As for the greens, you can use any mix of them. Don't overlook spinach, collards, chard, beet greens, arugula, and other leafy greens, as variety is key and too much of anything can be too much. Some people also find raw kale difficult to digest. Spinach is high in iron, for example; iron is a nutrient you want to get plenty of, especially if you're cutting back on your meat intake. (If you're growing broccoli, Brussels sprouts, or other veggies, you can harvest their leaves to eat in a salad on their own or combined with other salad greens, or sautéed.)

    3 cups salad mix, 1.5 cups wild violets and 1.5 cups kale or any
        leafy greens
    1/4 cup roasted pumpkin seeds
    1/2 avocado, peeled, pitted, and sliced

½ Fuji apple, sliced

Olive oil

Aged balsamic vinegar

Himalayan sea salt and ground black pepper, to taste

Place the salad mix in a bowl. Top with the pumpkin seeds, avocado, and apple. Drizzle on the oil and vinegar, and season with salt and black pepper to taste.

Yields 1 serving

Pasta Dishes

Creamy Mushroom Pasta with Red Mung Bean Fettucine

The other day, when I was out of town, I had a craving for a creamy mushroom pasta I used to eat before I went dairy-free. So when I got home to Nashville, I made it with red mung bean fettucine. It was *so good!*

1 tablespoon coconut oil

½ onion, chopped

6 to 7 medium baby bella mushrooms, chopped

1 teaspoon garlic powder

A few pinches flour

1 cup vegetable broth

¼ cup nutritional yeast

½ cup white wine

1 tablespoon thyme leaves, chopped

1 teaspoon tarragon powder

¼ cup coconut cream

2 tablespoons coconut water

1 tablespoon parsley

Vegan parmesan, to taste

Red mung bean or regular fettucine, cooked (2 servings, according to box measurements, or depending on how hungry you are!)

Heat the coconut oil for a minute in a large skillet. Add the onion and sauté for 5 minutes. Add the mushrooms and garlic powder and sauté 2 minutes. Sprinkle with flour and stir well. Add the broth, nutritional yeast, and white wine, and cook 5 more minutes. Add the thyme, tarragon, coconut cream, and coconut water. Cook on low another 5 minutes or until the sauce thickens to desired consistency. Sprinkle with parsley and vegan parmesan. Serve over fettucine, prepared as directed on box. *Yields 2 servings*

Paula's Bolognegeze!

My dear friend and fellow East Nashvillian, writer/director Paula Kay Hornick, adapted this recipe from her mom's "real meat" recipe, and now most of us request the vegan version because even the die-hard carnivores in our circle can't tell the difference! The last time she made this, my friends were afraid to tell me, thinking it was the real-meat version because it was too good not to be. But they were fooled!

Paula is happy to contribute this recipe. It's her famous "Bolonegenese," as I call it, or "Bolognegeze," as she insists is its real moniker. Whatever you call it, it isn't any ordinary Bolognese. It's crazy delicious and a fantastic way to prove that you can have all the flavor you'd expect from the best possible meat dish, with zero meat!

Because this recipe takes some time to cook, I recommend making enough to freeze and use later. It keeps in the fridge for three to four days too. Once you make it, you'll crave it over and over, like all of us "East Nasty" gals do now. It's also what I make to put in my zucchini lasagna, if I have time, or you'll find a much quicker (and less five-star cuisine) version of this under the lasagna recipe that follows.

2 tablespoons fennel seeds

Pinch red pepper flakes

1 tablespoon dried oregano

1 bay leaf

$1/2$ cup olive oil (1 tablespoon set aside to soak spices)

$3/8$ cup red wine ($1/8$ cup to soak spices)

1 medium red onion, very finely chopped

1 package Smart Ground "meat"

10 cloves garlic, chopped

$1/2$ teaspoon Himalayan sea salt and $1/2$ teaspoon ground pepper

1 tablespoon onion powder

$1/4$ cup grated vegan parmesan (plus more for garnish, to taste)

1 small can tomato paste

2 cups mushroom broth

1 tablespoon brown sugar or cane sugar

1-pound box of pasta (spaghetti or capellini; cook according to box directions, al dente)

$1/2$ cup chopped fresh basil, for garnish

Combine the fennel, red pepper flakes, oregano, and bay leaf. Add $1/8$ cup red wine and 1 tablespoon olive oil, and let the mixture soak while you prepare the other ingredients.

Sauté the onion in olive oil on medium heat until translucent, then add the Smart Ground (breaking it up as you put it into the pan) and $1/2$ of the garlic and cook another 5 minutes on medium. Stir in the fennel seeds/spice mixture, add the sea salt, pepper, and onion powder. Mix well and cook at medium/low heat for about 5 minutes, or until the meat starts to get just a little crispy brown. Add the parmesan and tomato paste, and mix together. Then add 1 ½ cups of broth, ½ cup at a time. Stir very well after each ½ cup, making sure to scrape all the meat off the bottom of the pan with each broth add. Mix the ingredients very well, cooking for about 2 minutes. Add the remaining red wine and the sugar. Cook for 10 minutes, stirring constantly, letting the mixture bubble and thicken. Add the remaining ½ cup of mushroom broth (be sure to constantly get the crusty tomato part off the sides of the pans).

Cook at very low heat for at least 30 minutes; get the water boiling for the pasta and time cooking it so that the pasta is ready at the same time as the Bolognegeze. Add more broth at the halfway point if gets too thick; cooking temperatures and pans will vary. Remove the pan from heat; fish out the bay leaf and discard.

Serve over your favorite pasta (Paula's favorite is capellini), with fresh basil generously sprinkled on top. Add a bit more vegan parmesan to top it all off.

Note: Be careful to use red pepper flakes, *not* ground red pepper!
Yields 4 servings

Stovetop Mac and Cheese (and Veggies)

I've been making various recipe versions of this for so long, at this point it's become second nature for me to whip up my own spin on it. This one takes a lot less time than other recipes I've come across. Bonus!

Cashew Cheese

½ cup cashews, soaked for 24 hours

1 tablespoon garlic powder

1 tablespoon onion powder

1 teaspoon salt

$\frac{1}{2}$ teaspoon ground black pepper

$\frac{1}{4}$ cup nutritional yeast

1 tablespoon apple cider vinegar

1 $\frac{1}{2}$ cups nut milk (almond or macadamia preferred)

Blend the cashews in a food processor for 45 seconds. Add the garlic powder, onion powder, salt, black pepper, and the nutritional yeast and blend for another 30 seconds. Add the vinegar and nut milk and pulse until blended.

Mac and Cheese

1 cup chickpea rotini

1 teaspoon olive oil

$\frac{1}{4}$ onion, thinly sliced

1 broccoli crown, chopped

4 to 5 mushrooms, chopped

$\frac{1}{8}$ to $\frac{1}{4}$ cup vegan parmesan

Cook the rotini according to the box directions, but shave 1 to 2 minutes off the cooking time. Heat the olive oil in a GreenPan for 1 minute, then add the onion and sauté for 3 minutes on medium heat, stirring frequently. Add the chopped broccoli crown, cook another 2 minutes, then reduce the heat to medium-low, continuing to stir. Add the mushrooms and cook another 2 minutes or so. Add $\frac{1}{2}$ to $\frac{3}{4}$ cup of the cashew cheese mix and stir to coat the veggies. Stir in the rotini and cook on low for another minute, or until everything is nice and warm. Add the vegan parmesan, turn off the heat, and stir until the cheese is melted. Serve immediately.

Yields 2 to 3 servings

Veggie Dishes

Basic Basil Pesto/Broccoli

I often make a pesto that I keep in my fridge when I'm home, as it's incredibly simple and delicious. If it's only me for dinner, one of my favorite meals is a copious amount of broccoli with just enough water in the bottom of the pan to steam it al dente, so that the water is nearly gone by the time the broccoli is done. Mix that with pesto, and there's nothing else I could want. Broccoli in quantities like that has protein and iron in it—not to mention a lot of water—so it's filling and great brain food, and the pesto makes it extra delicious. My dad's tip is to use the highly nutritious inside of the broccoli stalks in salads as well.

You can use pumpkin seeds or pecans instead of pine nuts, and parsley instead of, or in place of half of, the basil.

You can also turn this pesto into salad dressing! Simply put a generous tablespoon of it in a small bowl and add about 2 tablespoons of hot water to start. Whisk with a fork and add more hot water if needed until it's creamy.

> 3 raw cloves garlic
> 2 heaping packed cups fresh basil leaves (you can substitute
>   fresh parsley for some of the basil, if you like!)
> 2 teaspoons nutritional yeast
> 1/4 cup vegan mozzarella-style shreds
> 1/3 heaping cup pine nuts (or pumpkin seeds or pecans)
> 1/4 teaspoon Himalayan sea salt (more to taste)
> 1/2 teaspoon freshly ground cracked black pepper (more to taste)
> 3 tablespoons olive oil

Blend the garlic in a food processor, then add the basil, nutritional yeast, mozzarella-style shreds, and pine nuts. Blend thoroughly, and drizzle in the olive oil while doing so, if possible. Stop blending when the pesto reaches your desired consistency (I prefer it chunky). For a creamier pesto, you can also add a smidgen of water. Adjust seasonings as desired.

Add to your lightly steamed broccoli to taste—or to just about everything else!

Yields about 8 to 10 servings of pesto

Butternut Squash Roast

My dad has been making a version of this my whole life. My variation only has a few extra ingredients for bringing out the flavor in this delectable squash. It's about as easy and quick as it gets.

> 1 medium butternut squash
> 3/4 cup pecan pieces
> 1/4 cup maple syrup
> A few grinds of Himalayan sea salt
> Ground black pepper to taste
> Dash nutmeg, if desired

Preheat the oven to 350 degrees. Cut the butternut squash down the center, then scoop out the seeds. Place the squash facedown on a glass baking tray, very lightly oiled. Bake for 40 minutes. Flip the squash halves face-up, fill the center with the maple syrup and pecans, add the salt, black pepper, and nutmeg, and bake for another 7 minutes or so.

Note: This can be a side dish or a main dish, depending on what else you're making.

Yields 1 squash

Ginger Beets

I love ginger, I love beets, and they're both strong antiviral boosters. I put this together with ingredients I had during quarantine times.

> 3 small beets cubed (trim off any skin that looks blackened or bruised; you don't have to peel them completely)
> 1/3 orange
> 1-inch chunk of ginger, slivered, bruised skins and ends peeled off
> 1/2 Fuji apple, thinly sliced
> 2 teaspoons olive oil
> 1/2 teaspoon dried dill
> 1/4 teaspoon ground Himalayan sea salt
> 1/4 teaspoon ground black pepper

Preheat the oven to 320 degrees. Place the beets in a casserole dish or small roasting pan. Squeeze the orange over them. Add the ginger, apple, olive oil, dill, salt, and black pepper, and mix well. Bake for approximately 30 to 40 minutes.

Yields 1 serving

Herb-Roasted Potatoes

These potatoes taste equally delicious fresh out of the oven or served cold the next day with some nondairy sour cream.

> 2 Yukon Gold potatoes, cubed (skins on or off, your choice)
> 1 tablespoon olive oil
> 4 grinds Himalayan sea salt
> 2 healthy handfuls of fresh herbs: destemmed rosemary, oregano, sage, or dill

Preheat the oven to 300 degrees. Place the potatoes in a roasting pan, and add the olive oil and Himalayan sea salt. Stir to coat. Top with 2 healthy handfuls of the fresh herbs. Bake uncovered for 45 minutes. If you want to stir halfway through, you can; if not, the herbs will get crunchier on top, which is nice.

Yields 1 serving

Holiday Brussels Sprouts

This is from my post-Thanksgiving impromptu dinner I made for myself after our group Thanksgiving plans fell through on the actual day. I made myself a delicious feast on the Saturday after Thanksgiving, and this was the best Brussels sprouts recipe I'd ever made—perhaps because the pressure was off, since I wasn't trying to impress anyone. (Ernest is always impressed!)

> 1 tablespoon coconut oil
> 8 Brussels sprouts, halved
> 1/4 yellow onion, chopped
> Tarragon powder, garlic powder, and red pepper flakes, to taste
> 1/3 packet Beyond Meat ground "beef" (or substitute vegan bacon, cut into strips)
> 1/4 cup cooked chestnuts, chopped
> 1/4 cup dried cranberries
> 1 teaspoon coconut aminos

Heat the coconut oil in a large frying pan for a minute, then add the Brussels sprouts, onion, tarragon, garlic powder, and red pepper flakes. Cook for 3 minutes. Add the "beef" (or "bacon") and cook for 5 minutes. Add the chestnuts, dried cranberries, and coconut aminos and cook until the Brussels sprouts are tender/firm, another 5 to 7 minutes.

Yields 1 serving

Miso Eggplant

Miso eggplant is one of my favorite things to order at a Japanese restaurant. Since eggplant is so easy to grow in Nashville, I wanted to figure out a way to make something delicious out of it—and quicker than a lot of recipes I've tried, which require first marinating the eggplant or pressing all the water out of it.

> 2 cups eggplant, peeled and chopped (approximately 1 large or 2 medium)
> 1 teaspoon coconut oil
> 1 tablespoon white miso
> 2 1/2 tablespoons hot water
> 3 grinds Himalayan sea salt
> 5 grinds cracked black pepper
> 1 teaspoon raw agave syrup
> 1 tablespoon fresh parsley, minced

Grind salt into a stainless-steel frying pan, then add the eggplant and coconut oil. Cook on medium heat, stirring every 2 minutes or so, until the eggplant starts to give off water and begins to sizzle, about 6 minutes. While the eggplant cooks, whisk together the miso and hot water until it becomes a smooth paste and most of the lumps are out. Add the miso mixture to the eggplant, then the sea salt, black pepper, and agave syrup. Stir to coat, then cover the pan. Reduce the heat to low-medium and cook an additional 10 minutes, stirring every few minutes. Remove the mixture from the pan and put into a glass dish, add the parsley, and stir to mix. Add additional salt to taste. Refrigerate until cold if desired, or eat warm!

Yields enough for at least 4 appetizer portions

Quick Broccoli Coconut Curry

This recipe is perfectly calibrated to a GreenPan (see page 63), but if you don't have one, don't worry! Just add 2 to 3 minutes of cooking time to each instruction, and add a teaspoon of coconut oil along with the broccoli.

> Himalayan sea salt
> 1 broccoli crown, chopped into bite-sized chunks
> ¼ can coconut milk
> ½ teaspoon curry powder
> ¼ teaspoon garlic powder

In a GreenPan, add a few grinds of Himalayan sea salt, then add the broccoli and cook on medium-low for 2 minutes. Add the coconut milk, curry powder, and garlic powder, and stir to coat. Cover the pan and cook another 3 minutes, until the broccoli turns bright green and is tender but not overdone and the coconut milk is absorbed.

Yields 2 servings if eating as a side dish, 1 serving as the entrée

Black Bean Burger

I love black beans, and I love the convenience and protein of a vegan burger. But, delicious as they are, I don't always want to eat processed meat substitutes. Plus, unlike commercially available burgers, this is *extremely* inexpensive to make, proving once again that plant-based food doesn't have to be costly to be delicious! (At $0.99 for a 13-ounce container of organic black beans, I estimate the total cost of all the ingredients for this dish is around $1.50.)

> 4 tablespoons aquafaba (page 201)
> 1 cup black beans, drained
> 2 heaping tablespoons chopped pecans

½ cup chopped parsley

2 dates, chopped

1 teaspoon onion powder

½ teaspoon dried dill

1 dash chili powder

6 grinds of Himalayan sea salt

1 teaspoon coconut oil (or avocado oil)

2 tablespoons quick oats

¼ cup gluten-free all-purpose flour (for spreading on a board)

2 teaspoons sunflower oil or olive oil

Whip the aquafaba with an electric hand mixer until frothy. In a food processor, add 3 tablespoons of aquafaba, the black beans, pecans, parsley, dates, onion powder, dill, chili powder, salt, coconut oil, and quick oats. Mix only until combined but still chunky, about five or six pulses (do not turn into a paste).

Scoop out the contents, half at a time. Form into a ball and place on a board that's covered in flour. Turn to coat all sides. Turn again on the top and bottom, while flattening the ball into a patty. Repeat with the remaining half of the bean mixture.

Put the sunflower oil or olive oil in a skillet and preheat on medium-low for 2 minutes.

Place the burgers in the skillet and cook on medium/medium-low heat for 4 minutes. Flip and cook another 4 minutes on the other side. Flip once more, making sure the burgers absorb any remaining oil, and cook another 4 minutes. Press the back of a spatula into the tops of the burgers from time to time. Flip again and cook for 4 minutes, once more pressing into the tops of the burgers with that back of your spatula.

Yields 2 servings

Sea-Free "Crab" Melt

A nice side dish for this is sautéed spinach, cooked on low heat for five minutes with a dash of olive oil and a little curry powder. The extra warmth combines with this melt for the perfect comfort treat meal—and a well-balanced plate to boot!

> ½ teaspoon coconut oil, plus more for the toast
> 2 jackfruit "crab" cakes (Trader Joe's or other brand)
> 2 slices Ezekiel bread
> 1 to 2 tablespoons pesto (page 227)
> 1 to 2 slices vegan cheddar or gouda cheese
> Sliced avocado and papaya, optional

Heat the coconut oil in a large frying pan for a minute, and then cook the "crab" cakes on low heat, until nicely browned on both sides, about 10 minutes. Add a bit more oil if needed to prevent the cakes from sticking. Break the cakes apart into small pieces. While the crab cake cooks, toast the Ezekiel bread, then spread some coconut oil on one side of each slice. On the other side, spread a generous layer of pesto. Place a slice of the vegan cheese on the bread slice, followed by the "crab" and then another slice of cheese. Top with the other slice of bread, pesto side facing in. Cook the sandwich in the same pan on medium-low for about 3 minutes. (The coconut oil on the bread should be enough to keep it from sticking, but if not, you can add a bit more.) After the sandwich has started to melt and sizzle, carefully flip it over and cook on the other side. Serve with sliced avocado and papaya, if desired.

Yields 1 serving

Zucchini Lasagna

I love to make this, whether or not I have homegrown zucchinis that need eating, because it's just as satiating as pasta-based lasagna, but so much lighter. I'd describe it as "full but not about to explode." And if you've ever seen *Monty Python's The Meaning of Life*, you know the perils of feeling like you're about to explode.

Note: You can also make this with rice lasagna noodles (cooked as directed on box) or traditional lasagna pasta.

Fancy Tofu Cashew Ricotta

This needs preparation two days in advance. You'll find basic instructions for making a quick tofu or cashew ricotta on page 202.

> 1 package extra-firm tofu, drained
> 1 cup cashew cream (page 202)
> 2 capsules probiotics (I like Ora brand, but any will do)
> 1 tablespoon fresh parsley, chopped
> 1 tablespoon fresh chives, chopped
> 1/2 teaspoon lemon juice
> 1/4 teaspoon Himalayan sea salt, or to taste

In a medium mixing bowl, combine the tofu and cashew cream, add the probiotics, and stir well. Cover and refrigerate for 2 days. Remove from the fridge and add the parsley, chives, lemon juice, and Himalayan sea salt. Mix well and store in the fridge up to 4 days.

"Meat" Sauce

Here's my basic "meat" sauce recipe, which is more like a traditional tomato-y Italian lasagna sauce—in case you're not making this dish with Paula's Bolognegeze (page 223)!

Himalayan sea salt

1 tablespoon olive oil

1/2 yellow onion, diced

1 16-ounce package Beyond Meat

2 tablespoons fresh basil, chopped

1 1/2 tablespoons fresh oregano, chopped

Dash chili powder

8 grinds black pepper

9 ounces tomato paste (1 1/2 6-ounce cans)

1 1/2 cups low-sodium vegetable broth

Grind Himalayan sea salt on the surface of a skillet first, to coat, and heat for 30 seconds on medium. Then add the olive oil and onion and sauté for 5 minutes or until onion is translucent and fragrant. Add the "meat," break it up, and let it sauté about 2 minutes while you chop the herbs. Add the basil, oregano, chili powder, and black pepper; mix well. Sauté 5 minutes to let the herbs absorb into the meat. Reduce the heat to medium-low, add the tomato paste and broth, and stir to combine thoroughly. Cover and cook 20 minutes, checking and stirring every so often. Uncover and let the remaining liquid evaporate, turning the heat back up to medium, stirring frequently to be sure it doesn't stick, another 5 minutes or so. Add additional salt to taste.

Additional Ingredients

1 1/2 8-ounce bags vegan mozzarella shreds (approximately
   3 cups, plus more for top)

1/8–1/4 cup vegan parmesan (like Go Veggie)

4–5 zucchinis, sliced approximately 1/2" thick and cut so that
   each slice is roughly the same size and they lay flat, by
   trimming the oblong shape on the sides

Greens Mix

    2 cups chopped kale/spinach or a mix of the two

    2 tablespoons pesto (page 227)

Put the greens on the bottom of a medium saucepan, pesto spooned on top, on medium-low heat. Stir occasionally, till the greens are cooked down enough to where you can mix them all together and they're almost the consistency of creamed spinach, approximately 6 to 7 minutes. When the liquid has evaporated, turn off the heat, cover the saucepan, and set aside.

Assembly

Preheat the oven to 325 degrees. Use a deep 8 x 8-inch square glass pan. Try to find one that's 8 x 8 x 2.7-inch or you won't have enough room to cover the dish with foil at the end, and the food will touch the foil, which means the lasagna is sitting too high. If your pan isn't deep enough, you can still make the dish. At the end try to arrange the foil so it's not sticking to the cheese. Better still, I'd suggest investing in a Pyrex or other glass, or ceramic, lasagna pan that comes with an oven-safe cover. I'm not a fan of cooking with the aluminum foil directly touching what you're about to eat, if you can help it. Plus, if your foil is touching the cheese, it'll pull the cheese off when you uncover it.

Put a thin layer of tomato sauce on the bottom of the pan, then a layer of zucchini.

Layer the kale/spinach mix, then a layer of mozzarella shreds, then a layer of meat. Place another zucchini layer, then the ricotta mix, a thin layer of mozzarella, and another zucchini layer. Follow with the remaining meat sauce and another layer of mozzarella. Cover the pan with foil, trying not to touch the cheese on top. Bake for 30 minutes. Remove the foil, add an extra sprinkle of mozzarella shreds and the parmesan. Cook for another 10 minutes or so, until the cheese on top is well melted (keep checking; if it isn't quite melting, add a little more cheese and turn the temp up slightly, especially at higher altitudes). Let the lasagna sit and cool for at least 15 minutes before serving.

Note: If you want to make a larger version of this in a rectangular 13 x 9-inch pan, you'll need to add 50 percent more to all the ingredients—except for the ricotta, which makes enough in this recipe for the larger size. Or just double the ingredients, and you'll have enough meat sauce to freeze for another time.

Yields enough for at least six, more if you're serving sides with it

Desserts

Chocolate Mint Avocado Mousse

There's nothing better than chocolate mousse, says I. Well, except for chocolate mint avocado mousse, with the healthy fats of avocado snuck into it! Plus, it's insanely easy (and impressive) to whip up when you have someone dropping by. If there's any leftover, you can freeze it, as it tastes absolutely delicious thawed.

> 2 ounces 100 percent cacao unsweetened chocolate
> (if possible; just make sure it's dairy free)
> 1 tablespoon vanilla
> 3 small avocados or 1 large, peeled, pitted, and chopped
> (approximately 1 cup)
> 3 tablespoons raw agave syrup
> 4 tablespoons coconut milk (not low-fat)
> 1/4 teaspoon Himalayan sea salt

10 drops real peppermint flavor oil (such as Frontier brand)
    or 5 fresh mint leaves
1/8 teaspoon guar gum (available in baking sections)
Mint leaves, for garnish

Bring a small saucepan of water to a boil, and place a heat-safe glass or ceramic bowl on top of it. Add the chocolate and vanilla, keeping an eye on it as it melts, stirring to avoid sticking. Put the avocado in a small food processor or bullet blender. Add the agave syrup, coconut milk, salt, and peppermint oil (or fresh mint, if using). When the chocolate is melted, transfer it (using an oven mitt to handle the bowl!) to the food processor or blender. Add the guar gum and immediately blend until it reaches a mousse consistency. Spoon the mousse into ramekins or tiny glass bowls and chill. Serve with a few fresh mint leaves and some berries on top, if desired.

Note: I love the idea of using fresh mint, but the mousse *will* blend better and be more smooth and decadent if you use peppermint oil, so that's what I'd recommend if you want that wow factor. Just be sure to use real peppermint oil, not spearmint. Don't go making chocolate toothpaste mousse!

Yields 2 large servings in ramekins, or 4 servings if you use mousse as topping for berries or other cut fruits

Strawberry Trifle

This is something I often crave, since I used to love fresh strawberry ice cream, and it was something my dad would make from scratch. Later, when I started eating "real" ice cream, Häagen-Dazs Strawberry was one of my favorites. This is a beautiful dairy-free (and cholesterol-free) adaptation and incorporates fresh berries too. It can easily be made with any kind of berry you like or have on hand.

1 5.4-ounce can pure coconut cream, chilled in fridge at least 24 hours (Let's Do Organic is what I often use; you can order it online)

1 teaspoon raw agave syrup

16 strawberries, sliced

Turn the can of coconut cream upside down and open it. Pour off the liquid and set it aside. Put all the cream except for 1 tablespoon in a small bowl. With a hand mixer, whip the cream until it becomes the consistency of whipped cream. Combine half the berries with the cream, and put it in the fridge again.

Put the remaining berries in a blender, add the coconut water, the reserved cream, and the agave syrup. Blend till liquified and set aside until ready to serve. Divide the whipped cream/berry mix between two bowls and pour the liquid around it. Serve with fresh mint, if desired.

Note: To make coconut whipped cream extra fluffy, you can add a small amount of guar gum ($1/8$ teaspoon) and 1 tablespoon of powdered sugar to start with. Tapioca starch can also help. Sometimes, depending on the brand of coconut cream and how cold your fridge got it, you don't need anything else added. It also helps to chill your mixing bowl first, but this step isn't necessary.

Yields 2 servings

Snacks

Cilantro Hummus ∞∞∞

I actually intended to make this as parsley hummus, but because I store both my parsley and cilantro in the fridge leaves up, with stems in glasses of water to keep them fresh, I accidentally grabbed the cilantro instead! I'll blame it on quarantine brain, but it turned out even more delicious than parsley hummus. This is delicious with fresh raw broccoli and zucchini slices.

> 3 cloves garlic (Maybe less if you're having company—I can smell my breath as I write this!)
> 1 can chickpeas, drained (save the liquid if you can use it within two days to use as a substitute for egg in a recipe)
> 10 stems of cilantro (full stem and leaves)
> 1/2 lemon, peeled (keep the pith on)
> 1/8 cup tahini (or 1 tablespoon sesame seeds or pine nuts)
> 6 grinds of Himalayan sea salt
> 8 grinds of black pepper
> 1/4 cup olive oil

In a food processor, grind the garlic cloves first. Add the chickpeas, cilantro, lemon, tahini, salt, and black pepper. Grind only until chunky—otherwise it will turn to paste! Stir in the olive oil.
Yields 1 bowl o' delicious hummus that won't last!

Creamy Black Bean Dip

A friend of a friend of a friend brought a black bean dip she'd made on board a boat trip we were both on, maybe twenty years ago. I've never been able to re-create her recipe, but I kept trying to come up with my own, since I loved the idea of making something delicious and dip-able out of protein-rich black beans. When I happened upon this combo, I knew this was the one I'd be making from now on.

> 3 small cloves garlic
> 1 (15-ounce) can black beans, drained

1 teaspoon apple cider vinegar

6 cashews

8 grinds Himalayan sea salt

1/2 teaspoon tarragon powder

1/2 teaspoon onion powder

2 ounces firm tofu, drained

1/8 cup olive oil

1 tablespoon nutritional yeast

1 tablespoon parsley, chopped, optional

Cucumber slices and/or chips for serving

Put the garlic into the food processor first, and mince. Add the black beans, apple cider vinegar, cashews, sea salt, tarragon, onion powder, tofu, olive oil, and nutritional yeast (and parsley if desired). Blend until smooth. Semi-peel a cucumber in strips, creating alternating stripes for decoration, then slice. Serve with cucumber slices (or any sort of chip you like—plantain chips are also good with this).

Note: If you'd like this Paula-style (she always requests this with any dip), serve with an additional fresh-chopped garlic clove, a drizzle of olive oil, and another grind of Himalayan sea salt on top (especially if you're worried about vampires—this'll keep them away!).

Yields enough for appetizers for 2 to 3 (or a very satiating lunch for one)

My Famous Guacamole

This is adapted from my friend Dawn's recipe, which she gave me a couple of decades ago. Thank you, Dawn!

6 ripe good-sized avocados, peeled, pitted, and chopped

1/2 onion, finely minced

2 cloves garlic, even more finely minced

Generous handful of cilantro, finely chopped

One organic and non-overly-ripe tomato

Cumin powder, to taste

Generous portion of lemon pepper—much more than you think
  you need

Himalayan sea salt (or other salt), to taste

Finely minced jalapeño or chili powder, optional

Combine the onion, garlic, cilantro, tomato, cumin, lemon pepper, and salt, mixing well and adding the avocados at the end. (They start to go brown once they're cut. To keep them green, put the pit of the avocado into the guacamole until you're ready to eat, and then stir well.)

Note: You can double up on preparing all the ingredients except the avocados, and store that mixture in the fridge if you're expecting more people at a later time. Use half the mixture for the first batch, and when you're ready for round two, take the remainder out, add the avocados, and you're ready to rejoin the party (and everyone'll be even more glad to see you again than they normally are).

Yields plenty of guacamole for a party of ten!

Drinks

Until I starred in *Playing Mona Lisa* when I was twenty-three, I'd never had a drink. Because I'd had such an unhealthy relationship with food, I wasn't sure if that would translate to alcohol in the same way. Brooke Langton, who played my best friend in the movie, suggested I try port. I loved its sweet, desserty, decadent flavor, and I loved the tiny wine glass it came in, and that became a delightful routine when we'd go out to a bar. Plus, port is so rich, you really have to sip it slowly.

The first time I got drunk was during the week and a half I spent working on *The Sopranos* with Michael Imperioli later that year, playing the fabulously fake D-Girl of the episode's title. When I told him I was a classical pianist, he said he owned a bar on the Lower East Side in Manhattan, with a piano, and he'd love to hear me play. Some of the crew was coming by a bit later that Friday evening. Would I like to join them?

By the time I got there, I hadn't had dinner, and after a long week of work, I thought it would be a good idea to order a Cosmopolitan, another drink I'd only just discovered. That went down easy, so someone asked if I wanted another, and that went down easy too. On an empty stomach as a nondrinker. When I finally sat down at the piano, that was the moment it all hit me. I wasn't just buzzed: I was *drunk*. Not only was it my first time, but I also learned I cannot play classical piano in that state. Of course I chose a Chopin Ballade, the hardest piece I knew, because I wanted to show off, but it was like my fingers were one or two steps behind my brain. I knew what I was supposed to be playing, but my fingers wouldn't work. Michael had pulled up a chair and was sitting expectantly about two feet away from me, eyes fixed on the extraordinary feat he was about to witness. It was extraordinary, all right!

I spoke to both Michael and Drea de Matteo, who played Adriana, recently, and they both swear they had no idea. But Drea pointed out they were all pretty hammered, which I'd never thought of until that moment!

The Alicia Margarita

I have turned most of my partaking friends on to high-quality tequila as a substitute for wine, beer, or cheap whiskey. It is not only delicious, clean, and hangover-free (when drunk in moderation, and not mixed with crappy sugary mixes of course!), but it also has much lower acidity and sugar than other alcohols. And fewer calories as well!

2 ounces high-quality blanco tequila (Ocho and Casamigos are
  my favorites, but any clear tequila will do!)
1 ounce fresh-squeezed lime juice
$\frac{1}{2}$ ounce fresh-squeezed orange juice
$\frac{1}{2}$ ounce fresh-squeezed lemon juice (adjust these to taste)
Small squeeze of raw agave syrup
Ice cubes
Crushed ice
Coarse Himalayan sea salt or sugar, optional

Fiercely shake the tequila, lime juice, orange juice, lemon juice, and agave syrup in a shaker, with solid cubes of ice, until frothy. Pour over crushed ice. If desired, first rub the glass rim into half a cut orange, to coat with a bit of juice, and then dip the rim into a plate of either coarse Himalayan sea salt or sugar, if you want a salted or sugared rim.

When out at a bar, this drink can easily be modified: ask for silver tequila, shaken with pineapple or grapefruit juice, and served with fresh lime wedges you can squeeze into your drink yourself. The extra sugar in the grapefruit and pineapple takes the place of the agave.
Yields 1 serving

The Citrus Blast Margarita

With this version, you get the full nutrients and health benefits of these incredible citrus fruits.

Citrus Mix

1 orange, peeled
1 lemon, peeled
1 lime, peeled
$\frac{1}{4}$ cup water

Margarita

> 4 ounces citrus mix
>
> 2 ounces high-quality blanco tequila
>
> 1/3 ounce Grand Marnier or Cointreau
>
> Small squeeze of raw agave syrup
>
> Crushed ice
>
> Fresh mint for garnish

Place the orange, lemon, and lime in a Vitamix blender with the water and liquify (if you don't have a Vitamix, you'll need to strain the mixture after blending it). Add the mixture to a shaker with the tequila, Grand Marnier/ Cointreau, and agave syrup, and shake fiercely with ice until frothy. Pour over crushed ice. Garnish with fresh mint.

Note: I use 1/3 of the citrus mix per margarita, and store the rest in the fridge for up to 4 days.

Yields 1 serving

Cucumber Ice Cubes Are a Great Way to Save Fresh Cucumbers

This idea came from yet another one of my bumper crops, in 2019. One of my favorite tricks is to peel some cucumbers, put them in a blender or Vitamix, add a little bit of water, and blend well. Then I pour this into some ice cube trays and let it freeze. These cubes are a delightful addition to cold drinks—with alcohol or just to freshen up your water on a hot day. I also love to do this with watermelon.

Gin Fizz

I was in the mood for getting fancy with it a few years ago, using pine simple syrup leftover from a Christmas party I'd thrown—but regular simple syrup will do too. (You can also make your own even more delicious simple syrup: add a tablespoon of organic raw cane sugar and a tablespoon of low-glycemic monk fruit sugar to a few tablespoons of hot water; mix till liquified.) And I'm loving experimenting with aquafaba as an egg-white substitute, particularly in traditional cocktails that are made using raw eggs. I'd like to take this opportunity to point out that a friend of mine became severely, dangerously ill with salmonella poisoning and was hospitalized for an entire week after consuming a few cocktails made with raw eggs. So, even if you don't choose to cut eggs from your diet completely, I highly recommend not using raw eggs in cocktails. It seems to me that this is a chance to play it safe—and the drink tastes just as good, I promise. And then you can enjoy your eggs in dishes where you can really taste them.

    2 ounces gin
    1/2 ounce Cointreau
    1/4 ounce simple syrup
    1 ounce aquafaba (page 201)
    Solid ice cubes
    Crushed ice
    Rosemary sprig and green olives for garnish

Fiercely shake the gin, Cointreau, simple syrup, and aquafaba in a shaker, with solid cubes of ice, until frothy. Pour over crushed ice. Serve with a rosemary sprig and green olives on a skewer.
Yields 1 serving

Pumpkin Spice Martini

You'll find the recipe for my homemade nut milk at the end of this section. To make the pumpkin spice martini, you first need pumpkin spice milk. It makes the perfect welcome-to-fall cocktail.

> ½ cup pumpkin spice nut milk (page 249)
> 2 ounces gin, vodka, or tequila (I'm not much of a vodka drinker, but this recipe works well with that!)
> ½ teaspoon pumpkin pie spice
> ½ teaspoon ground cinnamon

Mix the pumpkin spice nut milk, gin/vodka/tequila, pumpkin pie spice, and cinnamon together and shake fiercely in a shaker with ice. Serve straight up with a sprinkle of nutmeg on top.

Yield 1 serving

Watermelon Rosemary Summer

Two of my favorite things, combined into a wonderful cocktail! I loved discovering that rosemary leaves blend with watermelon as well as they do. The juice retains its pink color because you don't need much rosemary to give it this subtle flavor. Rosemary is also anti-inflammatory and good for your brain, among other things.

> 8 big watermelon cubes
> 10 rosemary leaves, plus 1 sprig for garnish
> 2 ounces Bombay Sapphire gin

Blend the watermelon and rosemary leaves in a blender or Vitamix until liquified. To a cocktail shaker, add 3 ounces of that mix, and save the rest in the fridge (it'll keep for a few days). Add the gin and top with a rosemary sprig.

Yields 1 serving

Alcohol-Free Cocktails!

I enjoy spirits, but I also take at least two weeks off from partaking, at least twice a year. And of course, I have many friends who do not drink. A super-easy adaptation for creating virgin versions of pretty much all of the above: substitute equal parts aloe juice for the alcohol indicated in the recipes! (I like Lily of the Desert Whole Leaf Aloe Vera Juice for this purpose.)

Pecan-Walnut Milk

Homemade nut milk is incredibly easy to make as well as incredibly delicious. Pecans and walnuts are loaded with antioxidants and help raise your good HDL cholesterol and lower your bad LDL levels. Walnuts are an excellent source of vitamin E and omega-3 fatty acids, so they're extra good for your brain. Pecans also contain more iron, magnesium, zinc, and B vitamins than other nuts traditionally used for milk. Adding the sunflower lecithin means this milk won't separate nearly as much when you add it to a hot or cold drink—much more the consistency of store-bought nut milk, but way more delicious and decadent. The lack of separating also means it's a lot easier to froth up to make lattes. This is because the lecithin helps keep the good fats combined together.

Tip: Even store-bought nut milks will separate if you add cold "milk" to scalding hot coffee. The best way to avoid the separating is to add your milk first, and then pour your coffee into the cup.

6–7 pecans

6–7 walnuts

3 dates, pitted

3 cups water, room temperature

1 teaspoon sunflower lecithin

1 tablespoon vanilla extract

3–4 grinds Himalayan sea salt

For a Pumpkin Spice version, add:

1/2 teaspoon more lecithin

1/2 teaspoon cinnamon

1/4–1/2 teaspoon pumpkin pie spice, optional, to taste

2 heaping tablespoons pumpkin puree

Soak the pecans and walnuts in cool water in the fridge, overnight if possible, or for at least an hour or two, then drain. In a Vitamix or other blender, add the room-temperature water, pecans, walnuts, dates, sunflower lecithin, vanilla extract, and salt. Blend until liquified.

There's no need to strain the milk, especially if you soak the nuts first. Or you can strain in a paint thinner bag (available from online retailers) or nut milk bag if you aren't using a Vitamix and your blender doesn't quite whip everything all the way into a liquid. If you choose to make this milk with almonds, you will need to strain it.

Note: You can use one tablespoon of maple syrup instead of dates, if you don't have them handy. Also, you can store this milk in the fridge for three to four days.

Yields about 3 cups

PART VI

The

exercises

CHAPTER 10

Low-Stress, Small Changes Exercises

Clear as day I see the frame
beneath this steel
The empty spaces in the shape of you

—"NEW WORD"

I can't imagine life without a good daily (and short!) exercise session. This is a big shift from twenty years ago, when I'd come home from work and stuff myself and fall asleep. Now, if I have one of those grueling night shoots, I'll come home, meditate or journal, and breathe deeply in bed with some strategic essential oil combinations until I find sleep. Because now I know that I'm not hungry or particularly upset about anything—I'm just plain tired. If I don't feel tired at first, it's precisely *because* I am.

Exercise can be counterintuitive on one level because you might think, *I'm too tired to exercise,* but if you do start your body moving, you'll be less exhausted—and you'll absolutely sleep more deeply too. Working out will help you look better, but more importantly, it helps you feel better—which is the most important element of looking great (and staying motivated to keep working out).

When I was twenty, my job on *Cybill* afforded me the luxury of working out three times a week for several years with personal trainer Bobby Strom. He forever changed the way I exercise, because my muscle memory and core strength from that consistent training has stayed with me ever since. Over the years, I've used my education from that experience, as well as what I've learned from several other trainers—including one I worked with in Calgary while playing a firefighter/arson detective in *Blue Smoke* for Lifetime—to formulate the basic, everyday exercises I do when I'm not training for a specific role.

Each of the exercises in this chapter might seem like a small change toward physical fitness, but they'll pay off with big, big results. The more comfortable you become incorporating concentrated movement into your daily routine—even if it's just clenching your abs while you're waiting for the stoplight to change—the more comfortable you'll become pushing your boundaries, working out more, and seeking out activities that make you feel good and have great results for your body and health. Combined with smarter eating habits and consistent mindfulness routines, these exercises will soon have you feeling like your most fulfilled, authentic self.

Finding the Best Exercise for You

There is one general rule about the best exercise for you: do what you enjoy. If you don't find a way to get joy or at least a sense of respite from exercise, you won't want to do it! Some people like to work out on their own, and others like to be in a group. There is no right or wrong—only something that engages both your mind and your body to get the latter moving. Here are a few tips:

- If you want to join a gym, most offer a free or reduced pass to scope it out. See if the vibe feels right and what classes are offered. If a class sounds promising, try it. You might love it (or not!).

- Go online. Countless videos for every type of workout class I can think of are on YouTube and other websites. Whatever resonates with you will be worth a try. When I went to Whistler on a girls' trip from Vancouver, where I was working on *The Exorcist* and my friend Neve Campbell was working on *Skyscraper*, Neve introduced me to the world of twenty-five-minute workout videos. I was skeptical at first, but after doing one with her for fifteen minutes, I was dripping in sweat, and we were laughing hysterically. Every muscle was aching for days after, in a good way!

  These videos are a fantastic way to work every part of your body, with the benefit of a guided class and without you having to leave and attend one, especially when the travel time needed to make it to and from a class might make the difference between being able to do it or not.

- If you like a solitary sport, such as running, but don't want to do it on your own, see if there is a group for that sport in your community. Meetup.com has groups for an enormous range of interests. I personally love running but I prefer doing it alone; I listen to podcasts or audiobooks, or music that inspires me, and use it almost as a form of meditation.

- See if any of your friends are interested in a sport, a class, or a gym. If you make plans, it's harder to cancel when other people are counting on you. I love doing this when I'm not feeling motivated to attend a class or go work out at my gym, especially in the months in between acting gigs, when I'm making my own schedule. I often need the "appointment" of a designated time and a plan with a friend to motivate me to show up at the gym when I say I will.

- Hire a personal trainer for one or two sessions. If you work out in a gym, they can show you routines and how to use the equipment properly. Otherwise, you won't be able to take advantage of what's there, and you could injure yourself. It's well worth it. Take notes and let the trainer craft a workout routine for you involving free weights, available machines, and core strength. If, of course, you have specific body issues and prior injuries, you'll want to customize your workouts, and a trainer can help you do this.

- Make a great playlist. Listening to music not only makes the time fly by, but it makes you feel good and gives you a beat to synchronize your moves to, especially when you're feeling unmotivated. (More on this below!)

- Exercise doesn't have to be all or nothing. Too often, people work out for a few weeks, skip a couple of days, and are so mad at themselves that they give up for months before trying to restart again. Take it easy on yourself. It would be much better to commit to a tiny bit of exercise every single day, incorporating different aspects into your routine and seeing what works for you and your body, and gradually upping the time and intensity.

Get a Move On During Those In-Between Moments

- If you're watching TV, do some exercises periodically while you do. Keep a set of light free weights by the sofa. See if you can hold a plank for a thirty-second commercial. (It's hard!)

- While waiting for an elevator or standing in line, you can do butt/hamstring lifts by lifting one heel at a time gently behind you in an upward motion for ten reps, then do the other one. (Be sure no one is standing behind you!)

- Do squats when brushing your teeth.

- In the kitchen, stretch your calves while you're doing dishes. Do slight arm lifts while you're putting your food back into the fridge or pantry. I also do heel kicks while I'm washing dishes.

- Lift the laundry basket in curls when you're putting your clean laundry away, as you carry it from the washer/dryer.

Make a Great Playlist

Around five years ago, I realized that for some strange reason, most of my exercise playlist songs were sad! Now, I've always loved good sad songs, but there's a lot to be said for filling your spirit up with what you wish to attract, particularly while you're working up a sweat and your heartbeat and breathing rates are up. For me, exercise is almost a form of meditation. I made a conscious decision to start earmarking songs that felt full of the kind of love and the kind of life I wanted to have more of, rather than the songs of angst and ache that I liked, but that were about the sort of love story I didn't wish to have any more of, if I could help it. (I can't say that I haven't experienced heartbreak or disappointment since I made that choice—I wish I could! But I have noticed that I don't feel any sort of pull or draw toward those sorts of relationships any longer, and if I see harbingers of that kind of heaviness, I'm not attracted to it. That applies to romance as well as to friend connections.)

My (Nearly) Daily Exercise Routine

I developed this simple routine because I don't always have time for a full workout. If you do this on a daily (or even every other day) basis, I'd be willing to bet you'll soon see a difference. Doing one set of each of these exercises every day will only take you six to eight minutes!

When I started doing these exercises just to keep my muscles toned, it made a huge difference in ways I didn't expect. My back used to get tweaked often, and I'd needed to get medical massages as well as see a chiropractor for adjustments to deal with it. A physician also told me that if I did a few daily exercises to improve my muscle tone, my back and core muscles as well as the rest of my body would strengthen. So I started adding weight resistance to my exercise routine and have been consistent about it over the years. It's incredible how much more in alignment my spine stays now, and how strong my core has become. (And I still visit a chiropractor and get therapeutic deep-tissue massages, but more for maintenance and keeping my system running at 100 percent.)

These exercises were a small change from what I was already doing, because I don't have time to go to the gym every day (and as we learned during the pandemic, it seems like a good idea to have an alternative to being in a gym or a yoga class surrounded by other people's heavy breathing). If I have thirty minutes to work out, instead of taking a quick run or using the elliptical machine, I'll spend fifteen minutes on cardio and the rest of the time using free weights for strength training. The more toned muscle mass you have, the more calories you burn, even when you're at rest.

You can easily do these exercises while watching TV if you like, or during commercial breaks. Or while you're waiting for your food to cook. You can even do them using something other than hand weights, such as a couple of cans of food, or water bottles if you're in a hotel room. The idea is to have something in your hands to add a bit of weight. The other thing that's great about a routine made of free weights is that you can almost always find a bench and a set of dumbbells at any hotel gym, no matter how basic its fitness facilities are. But you don't even need a bench to do these if you don't have one—just invest in a couple of sets of hand weights. They're inexpensive and don't need replacing. I've had mine for twenty years!

Always start with a light weight—with whatever feels like almost nothing to you, even if it's as light as two pounds. It's always better to have perfect form with a low weight than to strain a muscle with one that's too heavy. Even though I've been doing these exercises for years, there are days when, for whatever reason, I'm feeling sore or strained somewhere, and I'll go down to eight or even five pounds on certain exercises. (I usually use ten- or twelve-pound weights.) Plus, some days you will have spent five hours pulling weeds or running after the kids, so you can skip the weights.

As with anything, please always listen to your body. I'm not of the "no pain, no gain" school whatsoever. I believe consistency and doing the exercises properly is more important than how much weight you can lift. The goal here is to build lean muscle and improve your health overall.

Note for all these exercises: Try to do at least two sets of each of these exercises, even if you're starting out. The reason is that the first set will tear down the muscle a bit, and the second set will get even deeper into the tissues and tendons. If you only complete one set, you won't do much in the way of building muscle. It's best to do fewer reps, with lighter weight, and then move on to another exercise, and come back to the second rep, so you can be sure to feel (and see) the effects.

Lunges with Bicep Curls and Shoulder Presses

1. Lunge on your right side while holding dumbbells.
2. Do a bicep curl with both arms as you lunge. Return the weights to starting position as you come up from the lunge.
3. Start with 8 reps and build up to 16 to 20 reps.
4. Lunge on your left side while holding dumbbells.
5. Do an upward shoulder press with each lunge. Start with dumbbells at a 90-degree angle, parallel to your chest. As you lunge, move the dumbbells straight up, not meeting at your head, being sure not to lock or overextend your elbows. Move the dumbbells back to starting position as you come up from your lunge. Be sure not to lock your front knee as you come back to starting position.
6. Start with 8 reps and build up to 16 to 20 reps.
7. Do at least 2 sets; switch bicep curls to left lunge, and shoulder presses to right lunge.

Bent-Over Row

1. Standing while holding dumbbells, bend at the waist to an L-shape (not a U-shape), holding stomach muscles taut, with dumbbells straight down.
2. Raise the dumbbells to parallel with your ribcage.
3. Start with 8 reps and build up to 26 reps.
4. Do at least 2 sets.

Note: If you're at a gym with a rowing machine, you can use that as an alternative. As another alternative—or in addition to, if you have access to a bench—you can kneel on the bench with your left knee, putting your left palm on the bench, and, keeping your back flat, hold a dumbbell in your right hand and raise until it is parallel to your ribcage. Repeat on the other side.

Shoulder Fly

1. Standing straight, raise the dumbbells up to a fly position, then back down.
2. Start with 6 reps and build up to 12 to 16 reps.
3. Do at least 2 sets.

Note: I still can't do a full set with twelve-pound weights on these! This exercise is more difficult, and we don't use our side shoulder muscles in daily life, so please go easy on the weights, especially to start with.

Triceps Extension

1. With knees slightly bent in a light squat position, hold dumbbells at your hips, palms facing in.
2. Move both dumbbells backward, as if you're pouring water out of a bottle.
3. Start with 8 reps and build up to 16 reps.
4. Do at least 2 sets.

Dead Bugs

These are hard but an extremely effective way to work and strengthen your entire core. My longtime friend Bobby taught me these. We never could understand why they were called Dead Bugs though. Shouldn't they be "Beetle Flipped on Its Back" or, at the very least, "Dying Bugs"? A dead bug wouldn't be able to do this, after all. Don't be a dead bug!

1. On a mat or a well-cushioned floor (you don't want carpet burns on your back), lie on your back with your arms extended in front of your shoulders. Bend your hips and knees to a 90-degree angle.
2. Tighten your abs and slowly extend your left leg toward the floor, while bringing your right arm straight up, fingers pointing to the sky.
3. Repeat on the opposite side. One completion of each side equals one rep.
4. Start with 10 reps on each side and build up to 64 reps.

Firm Your Butt While You Brush Your Teeth!

Here's one of my favorite hacks: do your squats while brushing your teeth! You should be able to get about thirty of them in, each time. Be sure to go slowly and with proper form (below). If you brush your teeth twice a day, this will firm and lift your butt, hamstrings, and quads in no time.

1. Stand with your feet about shoulder width apart, toes straight ahead or slightly pointed toward each other. Be sure you have solid footing—no wet floor or slippery socks. If you're standing on a mat, please be sure it's secure before proceeding. I prefer to do this either with bare feet or in shoes.
2. I like to have one arm raised (the one you don't use to brush your teeth) so it's at a diagonal line up from the floor when you're lowering yourself to the squat position, like an extension of your head. This keeps your spine straighter—aim for a straight(ish) line from the lowest vertebrae

to the top of your neck, which in a squat position means the line points straight on a slight diagonal. You don't want to be curving your spine in a U shape more than you need to, as that puts strain on the lower lumbar. The raised arm helps to send your attention out the top of your head, even as you're squatting and working the hamstrings and glutes.

3. Feel your hamstrings working as you come up out of each squat. Push into your heels as you go.

4. Do reps until you're done brushing your teeth. For me this is usually 30 reps, depending on how quickly I do each rep. This also helps you make sure to thoroughly brush!

Note: If you have a bad back, hip issues, or vertigo, do these very slowly and carefully. If you feel any twinges, stop right away.

Optional: Side Lifts

This is great for your side stomach muscles, but be careful not to bounce as you come up. Smooth and steady movements, as with all of these exercises, is key. Start with light weights, and there's no need to increase to weights that are challenging for you on this one. It's more for toning than building a muscle.

1. Stand straight, with your feet firmly planted on the ground and a light dumbbell in each hand.

2. With slow, controlled movements and your belly firmly tucked in, extend your left side toward the ground, head continuing to face forward. Stand up straight again, then extend your right side toward the ground, and so on.

3. Once you've completed both sides, that equals 1 rep. Start with 6 reps and build up to 16.

4. Do 2 sets.

Broom Twists

This is great for your back. If you have a broom or something like that handy, you can hold it straight out in front of you, palms facing downward, and slowly pivot your waist from left, as far as you're comfortable going, to right, and back again. Don't swing or overextend—the key is moving slowly and smoothly.

A Few More Exercises with an Exercise Ball

Another inexpensive and useful thing to own is a big, round, and bouncy exercise ball. (Don't confuse it with a medicine ball, which is also a useful tool but is small and weighted, usually starting at ten pounds.) You can use it both as a makeshift bench for seated arm exercises or as a back support for modified crunches. While lying on a mat, you can also use the ball to do hamstring/glute curls.

Chest Fly

This is great for firming that stubborn little place we all seem to have in our armpit area, ladies!

1. Lie on the exercise ball, supporting your mid-upper back and neck, with feet planted on the ground and glutes firmly tucked.
2. Take a weight in each hand, fists facing each other. Stretch your arms out, away from your chest, and inhale. In smooth movements, bring the weights back to center as you exhale.
3. Repeat 8 times to start and build up to 16 reps.
4. Do at least 2 sets.

Chest Press

1. Lie on the exercise ball, with your head flat on the ball, supporting your mid-upper back and neck, with feet planted on the ground and glutes firmly tucked.
2. Take a weight in each hand, fists facing straight in front of you and elbows at your ribcage. As you exhale, bring the weights straight up (no need to bring the weights in front of your body to meet—this can build tension where you don't need it). Inhale, bringing the elbows back to starting position.
3. Repeat 8 times to start and build up to 16 to 24 reps.
4. Do at least 2 sets.

Glute Curl

1. Lie flat on a mat or a well-cushioned floor/carpet. Place the exercise ball under your feet. Put both your feet on top and roll it until your heels are digging into the top of it. (You can do this with sneakers on or with bare feet.)
2. Place your hands at your sides flat on the floor or the mat for support. With your heels, roll the ball till you are raising your butt slightly off the ground (your back should remain mostly on the ground though). You should feel this in your hamstrings, quads, and glutes for sure! As with all the other exercises, start slowly and do this in smooth, controlled movements.
3. Start with 8 reps and build up to 25 or 30.
4. Try to do at least 2 sets.

Acknowledgments

This book would not exist if not for Todd Shuster at Aevitas. Thank you for thinking to ask me if I had a book idea, so many years ago, and for believing in this one from the get-go, and for helping me every step of the way to take it from a mere idea into an actual book.

It also would not exist without Karen Moline, my extraordinary collaborative writer, who turned my giant mess of concepts and thoughts and stories into chapters and structure. Karen, you have been such a joy to work with, and the back-and-forth of creating this book with you is one of the most effortless and seamless creative processes I've ever been blessed enough to be a part of. Thank you.

Huge thank you, also, to Andrea Fleck-Nisbet, Amanda Bauch, and John Andrade at Harper Horizon. From the moment we met, I hoped and prayed you'd be the ones to bring *Small Changes* into the world, and I'm so thankful to you for believing in me, and in this concept, and being the best possible teammates for this first-time author.

There are so many dear friends who have directly and indirectly influenced this book for years, but I want to specifically thank my loved ones Eliza Ann, Paula, Melissa, Vanessa, and Fran for being my touchstones and frequent accidental taste testers and keeping me feeling grounded and giving me confidence while I was writing this book. You are the best cheerleaders a gal could dream of. Thank you to my beloved Ernest for patiently sitting with me as I wrote, keeping me company, as always. Thank you to my mom and dad, Bob and Diane Witt, my lifelong number one fans and champions. I also want to thank Donna Britt for being the first professional taste tester (aside from my incredible friends) to check out the recipes and let me know that they worked and turned out delicious, and Tambi Lane for photographing the food I dreamed up. And thank you to my friend Travis Commeau, for so beautifully, and peacefully, capturing me (and Ernest!) for all the rest of the photos in and on this book.

And thanks to each of you who read this. The notion that this mishmash I've collected over my journey so far could possibly help you make your own small changes is the greatest gift I could ever ask for, and I hope that you know how much that means to me. Together, I hope we can keep making a difference and learning—and I look forward to all the small changes we'll make, collectively. Thank you for being my teachers and my inspiration.

With love and gratitude,
ALICIA

Notes

Chapter 2

1. Mayo Clinic Staff, "How Meat and Poultry Fit in Your Healthy Diet," Mayo Clinic, November 19, 2019, https://www.mayoclinic.org/healthy-lifestyle /nutrition-and-healthy-eating/in-depth/food-and-nutrition/art-20048095; Daisy Dunne, "Interactive: What Is the Climate Impact of Eating Meat and Dairy?", Carbon Brief, September 4, 2020, https://interactive.carbonbrief.org/what -is-the-climate-impact-of-eating-meat-and-dairy/; David Branigan and Elaine Ruth Fletcher, "Eating Less Meat Essential for Food Security in a Changing Climate, Says New IPCC Report," Health Policy Watch, August 8, 2019, https://healthpolicy-watch.news/eating-less-meat-essential-for-food-security-in -a-changing-climate-says-new-ipcc-report/.

2. "Using Global Emission Statistics Is Distracting Us from Climate Change Solutions," CLEAR Center, UC Davis, June 26, 2020, https://clear.ucdavis .edu/explainers/using-global-emission-statistics-distracting-us-climate-change -solutions.

3. Transparency Market Research, "Animal Genetics Market: Increase in Meat Consumption and Demand for High Quality Proteins to Drive Growth," BioSpace, April 6, 2020, https://www.biospace.com/article/animal-genetics -market-increase-in-meat-consumption-and-demand-for-high-quality-proteins -to-drive-growth/; Rachel Nuwer, "What Would Happen If the World Suddenly Went Vegetarian?," BBC, September 26, 2016, https://www.bbc.com/future /article/20160926-what-would-happen-if-the-world-suddenly-went-vegetarian; Carlysue, "What Would Happen If Everyone Stopped Eating Meat?," National Geographic, Education Blog, October 31, 2016, https://blog.education .nationalgeographic.org/2016/10/31/what-would-happen-if-everyone -stopped-eating-meat/.

4. "They Eat What? What Are They Feeding Animals on Factory Farms?," Organic Consumers Association, accessed May 17, 2021, https://www

.organicconsumers.org/news/they-eat-what-what-are-they-feeding
-animals-factory-farms.

5. Tal Ronnen, *The Conscious Cook: Delicious Meatless Recipes That Will Change the Way You Eat* (New York: William Morrow, 2009), 48.

6. R. Alexander Bentley, Damian J. Ruck, and Hilary N. Fouts, "U.S. Obesity As Delayed Effect of Excess Sugar," *Economics & Human Biology* 36 (January 2020), https://doi.org/10.1016/j.ehb.2019.100818.

7. Susan Raatz, "The Question of Sugar," US Department of Agriculture, Agricultural Research Service, last modified July 24, 2019, https://www.ars .usda.gov/plains-area/gfnd/gfhnrc/docs/news-2012/the-question-of-sugar/.

8. Chia-Yu Chang, Der-Shin Ke, and Jen-Yin Chen, "Essential Fatty Acids and Human Brain," *Acta Neurologica Taiwanica* 18, no. 4 (December 2009): 231–41, https://pubmed.ncbi.nlm.nih.gov/20329590/.

9. Yanping Li et al., "Saturated Fat Compared with Unsaturated Fats and Sources of Carbohydrates in Relation to Risk of Coronary Heart Disease: A Prospective Cohort Study," *Journal of the American College of Cardiology* 66, no. 14 (October 2015): 1538–48, https://doi.org/10.1016/j.jacc.2015.07.055.

10. Mayo Clinic Staff, "Trans Fat Is Double Trouble for Your Heart Health," Mayo Clinic, February 13, 2020, https://www.mayoclinic.org/diseases-conditions /high-blood-cholesterol/in-depth/trans-fat/art-20046114; Meagan Bridges et al., "Facts About Trans Fats," Medline Plus, US National Library of Medicine, May 26, 2020, https://medlineplus.gov/ency/patientinstructions/000786.htm.

11. Rene Lynch, "Tal Ronnen Says Make It Vegan But Make It Delicious," *Los Angeles Times*, June 23, 2011, https://www.latimes.com/health/la-xpm-2011 -jun-23-la-fo-tal-ronnen-20110623-story.html.

12. "What Is It About Coffee?," Harvard Medical School, Harvard Health Publishing, February 14, 2012, https://www.health.harvard.edu/staying -healthy/what-is-it-about-coffee; Kathleen M. Zelman, "The Buzz on Coffee," WebMD, accessed April 1, 2021, https://www.webmd.com/diet/features /the-buzz-on-coffee#1.

13. "Spilling the Beans: How Much Caffeine Is Too Much?," US Food & Drug Administration, December 12, 2018, https://www.fda.gov/consumers /consumer-updates/spilling-beans-how-much-caffeine-too-much.

14. Alina Petre, "8 Health Benefits of Yerba Mate (Backed by Science)," Healthline, December 17, 2018, https://www.healthline.com/nutrition /8-benefits-of-yerba-mate.

15. Elizabeth Weise, "Sixty Percent of Adults Can't Digest Milk," ABC News,

August 30, 2009, https://abcnews.go.com/Health/WellnessNews
/story?id=8450036.

16. "Calcium," Harvard T. H. Chan School of Public Health, The Nutrition Source, accessed April 1, 2021, https://www.hsph.harvard.edu/nutritionsource/calcium/.

Chapter 3

1. Barbara Haumann, "How Is Organic Food Grown?," Organic Trade Association, accessed April 1, 2021, https://ota.com/organic-101/how-organic-food-grown.

2. "Dirty Dozen: EWG's 2021 Shopper's Guide to Pesticides in Produce," Environmental Working Group, accessed April 1, 2021, https://www.ewg.org /foodnews/dirty-dozen.php.

3. "Hazardous Cookware," Occupational Knowledge International, accessed April 1, 2021, http://www.okinternational.org/cookware.

4. "Is Plastic a Threat to Your Health?," Harvard Medical School, Harvard Health Publishing, December 1, 2019, https://www.health.harvard.edu /staying-healthy/is-plastic-a-threat-to-your-health.

5. Bahare Salehi et al., "Resveratrol: A Double-Edged Sword in Health Benefits," *Biomedicines* 6, no. 3 (September 2018): 91, https://doi.org/10.3390 /biomedicines6030091; Nayana Ambardekar, "Resveratrol Supplements," WebMD, November 11, 2020, https://www.webmd.com/heart-disease /resveratrol-supplements.

Chapter 5

1. Tom Levitt, "Why Some Farmers Are Ditching Livestock and Growing Plants Instead," HuffPost, updated August 20, 2020, https://www.huffpost.com /entry/why-farmers-ditching-livestock-growing-plants_n_5e9620b8c5b6a447 0cb77646; Nadra Nittle, "The Plant-Based Movement to Transition Farmers Away from Meat and Dairy Production," Civil Eats, January 13, 2020, https:// civileats.com/2020/01/13/the-plant-based-movement-to-transition-farmers -away-from-meat-and-dairy-production/.

2. Michelle A. Waltenburg et al., "Update: COVID-19 Among Workers in Meat and Poultry Processing Facilities—United States, April–May 2020," *Morbidity and Mortal Weekly Report* 69, no. 27 (July 10, 2020): 887–92, https://dx.doi .org/10.15585/mmwr.mm6927e2; John Middleton, Ralf Reintjes, and Henrique Lopes, "Meat Plants—A New Front Line in the COVID-19 Pandemic," *British Medical Journal* 370, no. 8254 (July 2020): 95, https://doi.org/10.1136/bmj .m2716; Kimberly Kindy, "More than 200 Meat Plant Workers in the U.S.

Have Died of COVID-19. Federal Regulators Just Issued Two Modest Fines," *Washington Post*, September 13, 2020, https://www.washingtonpost.com /national/osha-covid-meat-plant-fines/2020/09/13/1dca3e14-f395-11ea-bc45 -e5d48ab44b9f_story.html.

3. "Dairy Farmer Retires Cows and Moves to Ethical Oat Milk Production," Plant Based News, last modified January 29, 2021, https://plantbasednews.org/culture /dairy-farmer-retires-cows-oat-milk/.

4. "About Genetically Engineered Foods," Center for Food Safety, accessed April 1, 2021, https://www.centerforfoodsafety.org/issues/311/ge-foods/about-ge-foods.

Chapter 8

1. "The Trouble with Ingredients in Sunscreens," Environmental Working Group, accessed April 1, 2021, https://www.ewg.org/sunscreen/report/the-trouble-with -sunscreen-chemicals/.

2. "Sunscreen and Corals," Coral Reef Alliance, accessed April 1, 2021, https:// coral.org/blog/sunscreen-and-corals/; Maritza Moulite, "Is Your Sunscreen Killing Coral Reefs?," CNN, July 9, 2018, https://www.cnn.com/2018/07/09 /health/hawaii-sunscreen-ban-questions.

3. Gyan Yankovich, "The Important Difference Between Mineral and Chemical Sunscreen," Repeller, May 2, 2019, https://repeller.com/mineral-physical -sunscreen/.

About the Author

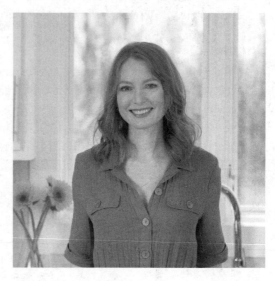

Alicia Witt has been acting since the age of seven, when she made her debut in David Lynch's sci-fi classic *Dune*. She was most recently seen in Netflix's 2021 hit *I Care a Lot*; other film credits include *Two Weeks Notice*, *Last Holiday*, *Mr. Holland's Opus*, *Urban Legend*, *88 Minutes*, *The Upside of Anger*, and *Vanilla Sky*. Her TV work includes *Orange Is the New Black*, *The Walking Dead*, *Nashville*, *Law & Order: Criminal Intent*, *The Mentalist*, *Twin Peaks*, *Justified*, *The Sopranos*, and *Cybill*. Alicia is also well known to Hallmark Channel audiences for her Christmas movies, many of which have featured her original songs.

A classically trained former competitive pianist, Witt coproduced her fifth release, 2021's *The Conduit*, with Jordan Lehning and Bill Reynolds. She has performed all over the world, including at the famed Grand Ole Opry, as well as opening for Ben Folds Five, Rachel Platten, and Jimmy Webb, to name a few.

Small Changes marks Alicia's debut as an author. She lives in Nashville with her rescue dog and copilot, Ernest.